AF700171

Nutrition for Women

Nutrition for Women

Ray Peat, PhD

Ray Peat Publishing
Eugene Oregon
USA

Copyright © 2024 by Ray Peat Publishing
All rights reserved.
Sixth Edition

No part of this book may be reproduced or transmitted in any form or by any means without permission in writing from the publisher.

Discounts are available for bulk purchases by organizations and institutions. Please contact Ray Peat Publishing for details.

ISBN: 978-0-9702913-5-6

Ray Peat Publishing
PO Box 5764
Eugene OR 97405
www.raypeat.com

TABLE OF CONTENTS

3. AGING

4. SOME DISEASES

5. PREGNANCY AND CHILDREN

6. DIETS

7. THE FUTURE

PREFACE

This book is intended for someone who already has questions about nutrition, or who feels insecure about the knowledge that is now available. I think it will answer many questions, while making you even more critical of the "official" attitudes toward health. Officially, women's nutritional requirements are not generally so different from men's. But all the special circumstances confronted by women in the U.S. haven't been considered by the compilers of official "Recommended Dietary Allowances." Some of these special circumstances that are important for women's nutrition are discussed here, with some general points that have sometimes been overlooked.

Since this book was published there has been a national conference on nutritional problems of women, and there have been articles and symposia on the nutritional effects of oral contraceptives. These "mainline" advances, however, still haven't caught up with the results of research. My recent additions to the book are intended to broaden the concept of nutrition and to direct attention to what I consider to be the most important problems and possibilities for women.

Delayed reproduction is one of the "newer conditions" leading to new physiological effects in many women. Disease patterns are changing, foods are changing, and the professions — with their normal 40 year lag between knowledge and application — are not able to deal with most of the new problems (they don't even deal too well with the *old* problems), so we have to become our own experts, learning how to find and evaluate useful information, to have an attitude of personal responsibility for knowledge as well as for action. The ideas in this book have been described by some as the physiological side of women's liberation, but of course there are political implications here too: why should we give privileged status to a profession which commits millions of unnecessary hysterectomies or which waits until the last quarter of the twentieth century to determine whether surgery is the best treatment for acute appendicitis (it isn't), or to the drug companies which fabricate their safety and effectiveness studies out of thin air, and then hire academic shills to promote their products, or to the food industry which adulterates and degrades our foods with the false excuse that this is required for economical mass distribution? Instead of giving them a privileged status, their criminal acts should be recognized and treated as such.

INTRODUCTION

Occasionally, I read parts of this book to see whether I still agree with the orientation I had when I was writing it, and I see that it seems to be far enough ahead of the general culture that it has something useful for almost anyone. Rather than changing it, I will just add some new information that I have been concentrating on in recent years.

A note on salt: On page 127 I mentioned "too much salt" as a cause of water retention. That phrase was a lazy gesture recognizing common medical opinion. If you suddenly increase your sodium intake, your body will take a day or two to adjust, and during that time you will retain a little extra water, but after the short adjustment time, you lose sodium at the same rate that you take it in. Under the influence of excess estrogen, your body retains extra water, and it is your appetite center which should balance that water by making you crave extra salt. If you learn to avoid salty foods at those times (or if you take a diuretic), your blood can't carry as much water as when it has enough salt, and so the salt stays in the tissues, rather than being carried to the kidneys. Tom Brewer demonstrated the importance of eating enough salt during pregnancy, to maintain adequate blood volume. When salt is restricted during pregnancy, the inadequate blood volume doesn't carry enough oxygen and food to the uterus to allow full development of the baby, and the kidneys secrete a hormone to increase the circulation, creating a tendency toward high blood pressure. Following Brewer's research, I saw that extra sodium should help in other situations involving circulatory inefficiency. Premenstrual edema, insomnia, and even high blood pressure often respond very well to a little extra sodium in the diet. One of the most important effects of sodium is that it tends to spare magnesium, which is likely to be lost during stress and hypothyroidism. If we eat salty foods when we crave them, we are able to retain our magnesium more easily. Sodium also helps to regulate blood sugar, for example by improving its absorption from the intestine. There is even evidence that sodium can spare protein, since, if there isn't enough sodium to excrete into the urine to balance acids, the kidneys will waste protein to produce ammonium as an ionic substitute for sodium. But I think the most important point to remember is that it is essential for maintaining adequate blood volume, and that it is almost always unphysiological and irrational to restrict sodium intake, because reduced blood volume tends to reduce the delivery of oxygen and nutrients to all tissues, leading to many problems. The emotional tension many people feel when they crave salt is, in some cases, the result of increased adrenalin, reflecting a real biological problem.

1. HORMONES

HORMONES AND PHYSICAL STATES: Suggestions, instructions, and possibilities for the Improvement of life.

A. Estrogen and the organism.

When I have observed that estrogen does things to consciousness and behavior, as well as to the body, I have heard these responses: if you say submissiveness is hormonal you are setting the women's movement back a century; if estrogen interferes with memory, then why don't IQ tests show women to be less intelligent than men? and so on. First, I want to call attention to a hidden assumption, namely, that "biological is equivalent to genetic." That is not true, they are not equivalent, but geneticists have been remarkably effective in convincing the public, and the granting agencies, that biology is ultimately nothing more than genetics. A typical argument for that equivalence goes like this: "if you say that an organism is more than its DNA you are a Lamarckian, and possibly even a Stalinist, and those ideas were disapproved by Weismann, who cut the tails off several generations of mice and showed that it didn't influence the inheritance of tails." If you have fallen for that argument (which is repeated from grade school to graduate school), read Zamenhof and A.E. Needham (and their references) on the transgenerational effects of diet and environment. Genetics developed in a context of "social Darwinism", and still has an ideological bias: consider K. Lorenz and G. Stent.

Second, I want to point out that men produce estrogen, especially under stress such as starvation or alcoholism or liver damage. In a famine, men may even lactate. Third, on the question of IQ tests, Dalton has shown that women who are suffering from an excess of estrogen do worse in both mental and physical performance than when their hormones are in balance. Women are not distinguished from men only by having more estrogen, as many people (including doctors) seem to believe. Quantitatively, progesterone is the main female hormone, and progesterone improves brain structure and function. The primary male hormone, testosterone, has chemical and functional properties of both estrogen and progesterone; this combined function gives males a short-term stability (fewer goiters, migraines, etc.) but a lack of adaptiveness in the longer range (higher mortality in infancy and old age). The placenta is a central factor in the development of the brain, but there is very little known about possible differences between males' and females' placentas, and their effects on such things as the greater mortality of male fetuses and the greater variability of males' intelligence.

Estrogen does block memory, according to animal studies as well as clinical experience: many of the women I see (especially if they have used birth control pills, have had special social problems, have eaten a vegetarian or soybean-rich diet, and if they have lived in a cloudy region) have very poor memory and a "foggy feeling in their head." High estrogen during pregnancy causes fetal brain damage and retardation. Too much unsaturated vegetable oil during pregnancy has the same effect. Both of these interfere with energy production: wasting oxygen, altering the effects of thyroid hormones, etc.

Estrogen is the hormone for beginnings, a sort of biochemical eraser which can eliminate recently recorded information, restoring the underlying primitive capacity for growth. When we are threatened, by injury or aging, we need the capacity for renewal of cells. Estrogen promotes production of prolactin, a protein hormone, and its close analog, growth hormone. Ionizing radiation, aging, and oxygen deprivation all cause biochemical changes similar to those produced by estrogen. Excessive estrogen (and the prolactin excess it induces) can be dangerous. A few biologists are talking about a "death hormone" which appears in the pituitary at puberty — I suspect prolactin (or another estrogen-induced peptide) is the hormone producing the effects they see. In salamanders, prolactin initiates the process of limb regeneration. Various cancers depend on estrogen and prolactin. A variety of substances promote tumefaction, lump formation, growth without differentiation. Rather than being hormones of death, I think of these as "renewal hormones," hormones of potential immortality. Anything which produces tissue atrophy will tend to produce cancer. The important question is, what will induce differentiation and useful function in cancer cells? There are many substances which promote differentiation and oppose the effects of estrogen, and some of these have been found to be useful in cancer therapy. Among the substances opposing estrogen are dopamine and nickel, prolactin inhibitors; chalones, the tissue specific proteins which inhibit cell division (and possibly more ephemerally, the peptides of memory); the aprotic solvents, DMF and possibly DMSO; progesterone and testosterone; thyroxin and iodine; magnesium ATP, the stable form of the "biological energy" molecule; vitamin A, a protein-sparing nutrient which promotes differentiation, and vitamin E (and the closely related coenzyme Q, or ubiquinone).

B. Organism and environment.

What does it mean to be biologically integrated with our environment, or with our experiences of it? For one thing, ***it doesn't*** imply a closed perfect timeless system; everything evolves. We have enough integration and consistency that we can survive, but an essential feature of the environment is that it is open and unlimited. When our environment shrinks, when there isn't enough food, we can adapt, for example by replacing muscle with fat and by having small-brained babies (the brain is an expensive organ, energetically, though its efficiency increases with its expense). When our environment meets our needs our brains and muscles expand. The lower leg (like the brain) is a good indicator of environmental support: parents who grew up in a population which has atrophied-looking lower legs can have children with beautifully developed legs, when milk becomes abundantly available. Boas (1912) recorded first generation changes in head shape in the children of immigrants. Brain size is likewise very rapidly increased with a good diet (or, in rats at least, with a more interesting life).

The brain (and especially its frontal tissue) is like a window onto both present and past environments. It saves as much as it can of past environments, but particularly, it saves those aspects of the environment which seem favorable, which hint at abundance and possibility. The frontal lobes of the brain are like the mainspring of a clock: in "hyperkinetic" people, in some psychotic and some lobotomized people, the mainspring — the energy storing system — is broken or weak: the clock will tick only when shaken. The individual with a defective mental energy storage system might dash around keeping his mind stimulated, or it might be that coffee or other nerve stimulants will raise the level of energy to the point that quiet integration becomes possible. The persistence of attention from one situation to another makes generalization and discovery possible. Given a favorable environment, the passage of time leads to the accumulation of awareness, to the discovery of new aspects of the environment, new ways of living; it leads to doing things more intelligently.

This can be said in physical and biochemical terms: if a shrinking environment doesn't interfere, the passage of time leads to a brain state which is both more energetic and more efficient. Vital stains show that these energetic changes go with structural changes in the cytoplasm, such that high energy efficient metabolism occurs when the cytoplasm has affinity for oily dyes. When water is at a surface it is ordered or structured so that it loses much of its wetness; a bug can walk on it; it contains more heat (or is colder for a given amount of heat).

Water is unusual in its capacity for internal structural modification, and for its heat capacity. During cell division, muscle contraction, and nerve stimulation, there is a release of heat (followed by an uptake of heat as the muscle or nerve recovers) which cannot be accounted for by any known *chemical* change. Its order decreases with increasing temperature, unless order is introduced by other substances. (The brain has used and exaggerated these properties of water.) Biological and environmental influences can modify these substances so that the cell water undergoes a "phase transition," analogous to the melting of ice. Muscle contraction, nerve conduction, synthetic and secretory activity, etc., appear to be regulated by these phase changes. Cooperative, or holistic, changes of cells and tissues are easier to understand from this integrated point of view, than from the conventional molecular and atomistic viewpoint.

These changes in the "solvent," or the intracellular medium, will alter chemical reactions — by modifying enzymes and by "sequestering" classes of chemicals, much as the aprotic solvents, DMF and DMSO, speed and alter reactivity. Following these "solvent" changes, we should expect the chemical consequences to amplify or "institutionalize" those changes. For example, proteins could be modified to produce appropriate patterns of "memory molecules" and "endorphins" (protein fragments having actions similar to morphine) and chalones. Patterns of excitation become stabilized as knowledge, and as developmental modifications of tissue: growth and aging and their ramifications. An excess of estrogen, or other factors interfering with proteolysis, could block the capacity to experience. The difficulty of recalling dreams probably relates to this synthetic (non-proteolytic) parasympathetic dominance during sleep.

The accumulation of aspects of the environment in our tissue, modifying our tissue's functioning and its affinity for various substances, is a short-time analog for the general upward drift of evolution, and it has presently known and distinct links with inheritance: hormonal influences pass both ways across the placenta, and maternal efficiency determines the supply of nutrients — e.g., sugar — to the fetus. "Lingering modifications," transgenerational influences of the environment, are visible in a great variety of organisms and organs, but it is in the brain — the environmental organ — that these Lamarckian effects are so visible and so crucial. If we think of the organism as an accumulation of its past environments, we must keep in mind that the accumulation is always occurring as the residue of the past strives to grasp (and to form) new environments. We do not willingly enter and conform ourselves to an undesirable environment.

C. Stress and politics.

Stress will cause a rise in estrogen and a loss of antiestrogens such as thyroid, progesterone, and (in men) testosterone. Male apes who are bullied have decreased levels of testosterone, and this effect persists long after their environment has improved. The stress of subjugation seems to lead to an adaptation of passivity. Their passivity prevents further injury, but we don't know how stressful their continuing submission is. Hans Selye found that the adrenals are a major component of our adaptive system. In the first phase of stress, there is a shock reaction (with changes resembling those of estrogen dominance), with injury to various tissues. In the second phase, the adrenals protect the animal, and this protection continues until something is exhausted. By exposing rats to a preliminary stress, Selye found that he could induce adaptation to other, later stresses — a kind of immunization to stress. About 1957, psychologists noticed that a rat could "learn helplessness": if they held a rat until it stopped struggling, it would then die much sooner than a normal rat does when put into a barrel of water. They also found that they could "immunize" their rats against learned helplessness, by previously allowing them to experience success in a similar situation. The short-term learned helplessness apparently does something to block the efficient use of energy, so that the animal dies of exhaustion very easily, i.e., it has depleted one source of energy without mobilizing another.

Energetically, the estrogen-dominated metabolic state is less efficient than the oxidative state which is dominated by thyroid and progesterone (or testosterone). The estrogen state, like the rats' state of learned helplessness, is "parasympathetic," in the sense that many chemical balances have moved away from the mobilized "sympathetic" or adrenergic state. The estrogen state, for example, depresses blood sugar, while the mobilized state spares glucose by oxidizing fat.

Since the rats can be "immunized" against becoming helpless during restraint, by previously experiencing success, it seems that something more is involved than Selye's pre-conditioning. It seems to be the ***meaning*** of the particular experience of restraint that affects the animals' capacity to struggle. The perception of possibility, of a vista that extends convincingly toward a better future life, seems to modify the metabolic apparatus. Drowning rats, it happens, will drown before they discover the liberating possibilities. Successful struggle takes a ***little*** while to get organized. I suspect that life in a rat-box was an essential factor in those experiments, and that a life of reasonable opportunity would prevent such learning of helplessness.

Men can be habitually passive, and can also have an excess of estrogen, so I am not implying (when I talk about the estrogenic state) either that the male sex is necessarily the source of human oppression nor that women invite their own subjugation by a hormonal predisposition. I do want to suggest that the hormonal conditions for easy subjugation are alterable, within the individual, from generation to generation and that better social conditions can improve our physiologies. High estrogen traits can be both acquired and passed on to offspring, as discovered by L.C. Strong in his mice, and as confirmed recently in rats that were stressed during pregnancy. I also want to point out that, within some privileged classes, women as well as men seem to actively promote their own role of passivity, relative to their men, probably because they sense that their position (and their children's) is threatened by widespread social and sexual change. Of course, men of various classes also encourage their women to be dependent, but my point is that historical and class processes are involved, and must be understood by those who want to improve human relationships. J.W. Prescott showed that, in all the societies he investigated, an inferior status for women was associated with sexual repression, self-mutilation, mystical-religious attitudes, militarism, and a hierarchical class system. Prescott suggests a two-state system in the brain, such that people do all those unpleasant things when they grow up deprived of pleasure. Interestingly, forty years earlier J.D. Unwin, a Freudian anthropologist who (unlike Prescott) favored repression, militarism, etc., came to the same conclusions. Behavior affects the hormones, and hormones influence behavior. Life in a rat-box society makes brains grow smaller, and makes people do the things that maintain the oppressive conditions. Nutritional and hormonal social intervention can change this.

D. Pleasure and hormones.

The first time I took enough desiccated thyroid to make my heart speed noticeably, there was a pleasure pushing up from my abdomen through my chest, making me want to smile and laugh. When I have watched suicidal women using thyroid or progesterone, there is a transformation (under an hour with progesterone, a few hours or longer with thyroid) from weeping to smiling and laughing; they speak of unbearable pain being replaced by pleasure. Women who have had orgasms while taking thyroid have lost their sexual responsiveness when they stopped. A woman said, soon after she began using progesterone and thyroid, that, for the first time in her life she felt that her heart and abdomen were opening with feelings of love. Another said "thyroid is love." Since these women were using the hormones for problems that had developed gradually, over several years if not their entire life, the sudden change was dramatic. They had forgotten that life itself was pleasurable. Our culture doesn't explicitly teach us that life is pleasureless, though it does make life pleasureless for many, and it does teach that pleasure is worth less than virtue, utility, possession, etc. By improving life conditions (in many ways) the hormones of pleasure can have a bigger role in our physiology. I think the experience of pleasure (whatever capacity for pleasure there is) increases the ability to experience pleasure, but I don't offer this with much hope as a therapeutic approach, since I know of people who say that running to exhaustion makes them "feel good" — neither "feeling good" nor "having orgasms" has a clear meaning, at present.

E. Nutrition and brains.

In regions where most people die before the age of five, those who do grow up are severely malnourished, and have brains that are much smaller than normal. Studies in Latin America have compared brain size and neurological development in villages eating "normally," and in nearby villages in which pregnant women and babies received a small nutritional supplement, and have shown that head size (and mental development) can be increased by a little improvement in the diet. Animal experiments, as well as a recent study of Americans, show that this improvement could be cumulative, if continued into the next generations.

Additionally, when the mothers' general health is so poor that nutrition just during pregnancy can't overcome the lifelong deprivation, the use of hormones could keep the mother in good health during pregnancy, and act as a buffer between the fetus and the mother's metabolic instability. In some areas, thyroid hormone would be crucial. In every area, for a large percentage of women, progesterone can improve gestation. **Thyroid supplementation would cost only about $2 per pregnancy, progesterone would cost from $2 to $15.** The difference between a passive person with an 85 IQ and an independent person with a 130 IQ is very great; if all the children in a village could be so healthy, many aspects of the society would change. I suppose this explains why none of the people who give money for research or humanitarian projects has been interested in supporting such a project. With adequate support, many foods could be evaluated for their effect, positive or negative, on gestation and brain development.

There is a medical myth about large-headed babies being hard to deliver. When the pelvis is seriously deformed, there is a problem, but the fact is that very large babies are delivered with great ease when the mother is in good health, because the factors which support growth of the baby also promote elasticity of the mother's tissues. Progesterone is such a factor — almost a "chemical obstetrician."

It has been observed that the ratio of brain weight to body weight corresponds directly to longevity. The brain has a nourishing, trophic influence on other tissues. A stable, efficient brain is an anti-stress agent. The hormones of stress age various tissues, including the brain, and the collagen in connective tissue. Good nutrition, including the anti-stress substances found in certain foods, will simultaneously optimize intelligence and increase the healthy life-span. Congenital defects are increased by stress and poor nutrition during pregnancy, and reduced by good nutrition, hormone supplementation, and stress reduction. Even in rich cultures, protein deficiency, inappropriate exercise, and emotional tension will contribute to premature aging of the individual, and damage to the offspring.

F. Long-range order.

There is a continuity from the molecular level through our physiological states into our way of life. The properties of water, modified by biological substances and biological experience, allow a kind of physiological (and epistemological) unity which is unimaginable for the atomistic genetic determinists. The existence of long-range order in a liquid is now respectable, because liquid crystals are in common use for watch dials and calculator display devices. Long-range order is a principle of biological thinking which brings us into a new phase of theory. Succeeding in biology, this principle can help us to re-evaluate other events in the history of ideas about physical state. For example, it is now clear that Polanyi's adsorption potential was a fact, and Einstein and Haber were dogmatically wrong in their ideas about inter-atomic forces. Seeing this, we should question the many consequences of the same mistaken atomistic view, including Einstein's theory of photoelectricity, which attributed a corpuscular quality to light, because he "knew" that matter was strictly particulate without any of the long-range energy properties that were later demonstrated by Polanyi.

Biology is now approaching a time when it will be increasingly frustrated by the inability of chemists and physicists to think clearly about the assumptions they have made. A few physical scientists have begun to realize that concepts developed in biology can solve problems in, for example, the physics of absorption. Thinking about life, our assumptions should be fewer and less arbitrary than in simple sciences.

When we speak about "our mental state and our physical state," we may eventually achieve the concreteness and generality which a physicist has in describing, e.g., "the solid state," but this will be an expansion of physics, not a reduction of biology.

WHY PRESCRIBE ESTROGEN?

Millions of women with already high estrogen levels are being sold estrogen pills or injections, often prescribed as treatment for symptoms known to result from excess estrogen. When this treatment fails, and symptoms get worse, a tranquilizer is often added to the treatment. Surgery frequently follows. Many healthy wombs are removed as a "preventive" measure. I have talked to many women who have been ravaged by this kind of medical treatment; asking them how their "low estrogen" had been diagnosed, they say "by a Pap smear," or "he could tell by looking at my eyes," or even vaguer methods. I have only talked to one woman who had her blood estrogen level actually measured.

Controlled scientific studies don't play much of a role in the practice of medicine. This widespread use of estrogen is not only unsupported by such valid studies, but is in opposition to most of the real data that exist. Foreign physicians have asked how it was possible to speak of "hormone replacement therapy," when the estrogen level in the blood was often maintained at 1000 percent of normal.

Hepatitis and other liver problems are known to be increasing. Women's livers are known to be more sluggish than men's in removing chemicals from the body. When the liver doesn't remove estrogen from the body rapidly enough, estrogen accumulates in the body — this is why male alcoholics often grow breasts. Estrogen pills and tranquilizers add to the liver's burden. Poor nutrition makes it impossible for the liver to function properly.

It has been known for several decades that many of the symptoms of hormone imbalance can be relieved with simple nutritional therapy. If doctors don't want to take the time to study the literature, they should at least be referred to one of the simply written articles, such as Biskind's on the liver and hormones in ***Vitamins and Hormones***, 1946.

SOME SYMPTOMS OF ESTROGEN EXCESS

In a recent nutrition class, a young woman who prepared nutritionally perfect meals (even exceeding the established "recommended daily allowances") was getting ready to have breast surgery, because for two years she had had painful cysts. One of the things we discussed was a 1946 paper by Biskind on estrogen and the liver, in which it was pointed out that a B vitamin deficiency slows the liver's elimination of estrogen, so that it accumulates in the body, producing a series of classical symptoms, including cystic mastitis.

During the course, we had also discussed how vitamin A can often benefit secretory tissues, such as the glands which maintain hormonal balance.

The last day of class, she told me that, for the first time in two years she had no breast pain, and her doctor had told her she was completely free of the cystic condition, and called off the surgery.

The other symptoms mentioned by Biskind include adrenal cortex hypertrophy, uterine bleeding, premenstrual tension, diminished libido and impotence in the male and cutaneous vascular spiders. He mentions that the diminished testicular function of diabetes can be improved by nutrition, as can an enlarged liver, and that PABA sometimes improves the libido. He wrote that thiamine and riboflavin seemed to be responsible for the liver's regulation of estrogen, but that the amino acid methionine was also essential. Lipschutz (Steroids and Tumors, 1950) reported that protein is crucial for estrogen removal. Recent studies in monkeys show that menstruation is brought on when the progesterone level falls and the uterine blood vessels dilate, then go into spasm. Many of the symptoms of estrogen excess are equivalent to those of a progesterone deficiency. Progesterone is a direct antagonist of estrogen; Lipschutz (and Korenchevsky) have shown that progesterone causes regression of tumors induced by estrogen. Thyroid hormone and Vitamin A promote protein metabolism and antagonize some of estrogen's effects. In fact, hyperthyroidism is known to be able to cause estrogen levels to fall below normal. Vitamins C and E are also known to help the liver deal with toxins. Puffiness, usually most noticeable in the face in the morning and the feet at night, is another common symptom of estrogen excess, caused by the retention of water and sodium.

ESTROGEN AND SEX

Masters, the sex researcher, recently mentioned that quite a few women have been losing their ability to have an orgasm after being on the pill for 18 months or longer, and that they are also losing their interest in sex, or their ability to be aroused easily. Since this doesn't happen to everyone, and takes a fairly long time to develop. We can probably understand it best by considering other effects of the pill that develop slowly. It's well known that taking estrogen can cause the blood to clot too easily. Other effects include anemia, low blood sugar, and slow functioning of the liver.

Some people will say that the pill inhibits estrogen production, and that the loss of sex interest means that these women need more estrogen. However, the other effects produced by the pill are pretty clearly the result of an excess of estrogen, at least in relation to other hormones. And I think it might be dangerous to increase the dosage of estrogen hoping to restore normal sexual function.

Normally, the liver treats estrogen like a poison, removing it immediately from the body. If the liver gets sluggish from malnutrition or too much estrogen (or other damage), it can allow the hormone to build up to very high levels. Since estrogen is metabolically antagonistic to progesterone and testosterone, I think the pill might decrease libido by counteracting these other hormones. They raise the energy charge of cells, and contribute to a sense of well-being. Testosterone stimulates sexual desire in both sexes. The energy charge of cells can govern nerve reflexes, and so I think it is reasonable to suppose that the quality of sexual arousal and orgasm could be influenced by the relative balance of estrogen and progesterone or testosterone.

An I.U.D. (intra-uterine contraceptive device) is known to be "luteolytic", meaning it suppresses progesterone formation and leads to a relative excess of estrogen. This suggests that I.U.D.s might also eventually make it hard to have orgasms. Copper seems to be synergic with estrogen, and could have a similar effect — could this have something to do with the de-emphasis of sex among some vegetarians who eat lots of copper-rich soy beans? Copper I.U.D's would seem the most likely kind to interfere with sexual satisfaction.

My impression (from women I have known) is that excessive estrogen will first produce little orgasms, with a need to have many in succession. The low blood sugar resulting from high estrogen can cause depression, irritability and sleep problems. When a lower ratio of estrogen to the other hormones exists, I think the pattern is more likely to be one large, intense orgasm followed by sleep, with the next arousal not coming for about 1 and one half hours.

If a person (especially, though not necessarily, a woman) has unsatisfying orgasms, or no orgasms at all, I think it would be advisable to eliminate the possible causes of a hormone imbalance (including high copper intake), and also to help the liver function as effectively as possible by getting good nutrition. High protein, all the B vitamins, vitamins A,C, and E, and zinc and magnesium are especially important. Vitamin E does several things biochemically which are exactly the opposite of what estrogen does, so it has been called the "anti-estrogenic vitamin."

Magnesium has a very powerful sedative — even anesthetic — effect, which seems to be especially favorable to healthy sexuality. I suspect that it will eventually be known as an "antiestrogenic mineral," and, with zinc, may turn out to be effective in a wide variety of sex-related problems. It is already a traditional therapy for prostatitis. Male impotence as well as female sex problems can sometimes benefit from special nutrition.

According to S. Zuckerman (1955), excess estrogen causes enlargement of the prostate in dogs. More recent studies have used progestins to relieve prostate enlargement in men. These observations suggest that excess estrogen may be a frequent factor in male sexual problems. I now suspect low thyroid is a factor in most such cases, and advise the elimination of nuts, beans, broccoli, corn oil, and other thyroid inhibitors from the diet.

VITAMIN E AND SEX

In another section on estrogen, I mention that too much estrogen seems to interfere with sexual responsiveness and orgasm, and I suggested that a tendency to have a series of small or only partly satisfying orgasms could result from an excess of either estrogen or copper, since copper and estrogen have some biochemical similarities and interactions. While zinc can counteract copper, many of the effects of estrogen can be offset by vitamin E. (Vitamin C can also detoxify and help to excrete metals.)

Estrogen seems to increase the body's need for vitamin E, as it does for many other nutrients. Pregnancy, which can leave the woman with an elevated estrogen level, seems to raise the amount of vitamin E needed to sustain the following pregnancy, if we can generalize from animal experiments. During the first year of a rat's life, the amount of vitamin E needed to sustain pregnancy increases by about 65 times (J. of Clinical Nutrition, Sept. 1974).

Just as too much estrogen causes sterility, it seems that it can also cause loss of sexual "capacity". Since vitamin E can often restore fertility (e.g.. E.V. Shute, J. Endocr. 2, p.173, 1940), it is likely that it can also sometimes restore the libido.

Newborn rodents often respond to stimulation with the behavior of a mature female in heat, and this doesn't seem to be produced by estrogen. Rather, it seems to be produced by the slight oxygen deprivation at birth. My own experiments have shown that vitamin E tends to raise the oxygen content of tissues, at least when the tissue is under the influence of estrogen. I suspect that estrogen acts largely through its effect on oxygen metabolism — a sort of biochemical breath-holding. For certain nerve systems, both taking vitamin E and having an orgasm might be compared to taking a good deep breath.

To continue the analogy between breathing and orgasm, having an orgasm without enough vitamin E would be like sneezing without first inhaling. Some people really do this, and the effect is a series of very small, quick sneezes. That is, if the nerve-muscle system can't get into the "ready state" the tension can't resolve itself normally. (This "ready state" of the tissues has been studied in the Soviet Union more than in the U.S.; I describe these studies in my book ***Mind and Tissue*).**

Vitamin E preserves ATP; ATP is a source of biological energy, but it also stabilizes or relaxes tissue. This energized relaxation is the "ready state." In a dead animal, ATP disappears from the tissues and the muscles contract and harden, but if ATP is injected the muscles will become soft again. In a vitamin E deficiency, certain tissues lose enough ATP that they can't function normally. Muscles cramp, and eventually can harden and become dystrophic. Magnesium also helps to maintain ATP levels, and for example can be used to stop menstrual cramps. In an extreme case of vitamin E deficiency, reflexes become abnormal; in some animals, softening of the brain is the first symptom of a vitamin E deficiency.

The highest part of the brain, in evolution, is the expectancy/planning system in the frontal lobes. Delayed and appropriate response is impossible if these lobes don't function well. In a healthy animal, arousal means expectation: the longer arousal can be sustained without distraction, the higher the energy charge will be, and the more intense and satisfying the completion will be.

Trying to sustain excitement too long, for example while waiting for your partner to finish an elaborate preparatory ritual, can exhaust the desire, the emotion and tension; the expectancy pattern fades. Losing sleep, or getting too hungry can have the same effect by causing low blood sugar. The brain needs a large supply of glucose to function well. Incidentally, oversleeping can cause the blood sugar to fall. High estrogen can also cause low blood sugar.

People have always suspected that sexual desire was part of the highest human functioning. The expectancy process in the most uniquely human part of the brain is as essential for good sex as it is for good art or good science. Adequate nutrition, including vitamin E, is extremely important for the full functioning of this system.

ESTROGEN AND THYROID: A NOTE FOR PHYSICIANS

The idea of physiological compensation is sometimes overlooked in interpreting endocrine interactions, with confusing results. The brain-pituitary system (not just the hypothalamus, since the whole brain and sensory system participates as "reflex setter") is probably the main regulatory or compensating system. If estrogen is injected into an animal, the level of thyroid stimulating hormone rises (Brown-Grant, *J. Endocr.* 35, 263, 1966). This should be taken as a hint that the peripheral effect of estrogen can be compensated for by thyroxin. If thyroid functioning is borderline, it would also suggest that elevated estrogen might be uncompensated peripherally. There are many known examples of metabolic or functional opposition of estrogen and thyroid.

Blood Sugar

Estrogen lowers blood sugar by stimulating insulin release (Goodman and Hazelwood, *J. Endocr. 62,* 439, 1974), and also apparently by blocking the synthesis of adrenal corticoids (Turner, *General Endocrinology,* Sanders Co., Phila., 1966), while thyroxin raises blood sugar (Turner, ibid.).

Fat Synthesis/ Lipolysis

Synthesis of lipids is promoted by estrogen (Peat and Soderwall, *Physiol. Chem. and Physics 4(3),* 295, 1972), while thyroxin promotes lipolysis possibly acting through adrenalin (Turner, op. cit.).

Liver Catalase Activity

Reflecting an altered respiratory pattern, liver catalase activity seems to be lowered by estrogen (Adams, *J. Reprod. Fertil. 12,* 9, 1970) and raised by thyroxin.

Proliferative Response of Lymphoid Organs

The proliferative response of lymphoid organs, measured as the rate of DNA synthesis, is increased by estrogen or insulin and decreased by thyrotropin (Maor, *et al., Acta Endocrinol.* 75(1), 205, 1974).

Size of Thymus

Apparently thymolysis is blocked by thyroxine, and promoted by estrogen (stress, radiation and starvation also cause thymus shrinkage).

Lactation

Starvation and injection of estradiol both suppress lactation while thyroxine injection stimulates lactation (Oshima, *Bull, Natl. Inst. Anim. Ind (Chibal) 26,* 45, 1973).

Opposing effects of these hormones are also seen in fever and thermogenesis, in fertility (Peat, dissertation Univ. of Oregon 1972; Harrison et al., *Principles of Internal Medicine,* 1950), and in methionine metabolism (Finkelstein and Harris, *Arch. Biochem. Biophys. 159 (1),* 160, 1973). (Brown-Grant, *J. Physiol. 176,* 91, 1965) has commented on the idea of compensatory cycling of thyroid activity: " . . . the sudden drop in thyroid activity during metoestrus and dioestrus could well be a compensatory decline below the mean level, resulting from the release of an excess of hormone above the needs of the animal during oestrus." The data showing peripheral opposition of the hormones suggest that the need for thyroxine varies with the estrogen cycle. The fact that myxedema is 5 times more frequent in females (adult) than male also suggests such an effect of estrogen (Harrison, op. *cit.,* p. 611). Water and sodium retention induced by estrogen (Korenchevsky, *Physiol. and Pathol. Aging,* Hafner, N.Y. 1961) may be hard to distinguish from the water retention of myxedema. Iodine, protein and electrolyte balance should be given special attention in women who may have an estrogen imbalance.

THYROID

Thyroid hormone is necessary for respiration on the cellular level, and makes possible all higher biological functions. Without the metabolic efficiency which is promoted by thyroid hormone, life couldn't get much beyond the single-cell stage. Without adequate thyroid, we become sluggish, clumsy, cold, anemic, and subject to infections, heart disease, headaches, cancer, and many other diseases, and seem to be prematurely aged, because none of our tissues can function normally. Besides providing the respiratory energy which is essential to life, thyroid hormones seem to stimulate and direct protein synthesis.

In hypothyroidism there is little stomach acid, and other digestive juices (and even intestinal movement) are inadequate, so gas and constipation are common. Foods aren't assimilated well, so even on a seemingly adequate diet there is "internal malnutrition." Magnesium is poorly absorbed, and a magnesium deficiency can lead to irritability, blood clots, vascular spasms and angina pectoris, and many other problems. Heart attacks, hardening of the arteries, and both high and low blood pressure can by caused by hypothyroidism.

"Spotting," "breakthrough bleeding," and abnormally long periods are often caused by hypothyroidism. In the light of this knowledge, I feel that a physician who advocates removal of the uterus for excessive bleeding, without first trying thyroid therapy, is not practicing medicine properly.

Low body temperature (below 98 degrees when you wake in the morning) and slow pulse are the simplest indicators of hypothyroidism. Foolishly designed blood tests have caused many people to be taken off thyroid medication, in spite of their symptoms. For 40 years, time after time one blood test has displaced another, and always the one which is in use at the moment is "the correct" one. The oldest test, the BMR, is still the best, in spite of the possibility of a mistake if the test is given when the patient has an infection, but the temperature is also a reliable indicator (except that heat from the environment — an electric blanket or a hot room — can artificially raise temperature to normal.)

Cysteine, an amino acid which is abundant in muscle and liver, happens to block synthesis of the thyroid hormone. When we are starving or under stress, cortisone causes these protein-rich tissues to be consumed. If metabolism continued at a normal rate, stress or hunger would quickly destroy us. The cysteine which is released from muscle, though, inhibits the thyroid, so metabolism is slowed. Cortisone also inhibits the thyroid. Any stress, including heavy exercise, will cause this protective slowing of metabolism. The slow heart beat of runners is largely the result of this adaptive hypothyroidism. When we eat large amounts of muscle meats or liver the high concentration of cysteine suppresses the thyroid. Heart, eggs, skin (gelatin) and milk are more favorable to the thyroid. Other anti-thyroid foods are peanuts, soybeans, raw cabbage, radishes, broccoli, cauliflower, unsaturated oils (such as safflower, corn, cottonseed, and soy oils), and an excess of iodine. Amygdalin (nitrilosides, laetrile) which occurs in many nuts, seeds and grains, is also a thyroid inhibitor. Because iodate is used as a "dough conditioner" (to make bread water-heavy), the American eater often gets ten times more iodine than is recommended. Combined with unsaturated oils, as organic iodides, excess iodine can powerfully inhibit the thyroid. Manganese is needed to synthesize thyroxin, so a deficiency can interfere with thyroid function (coffee is a major source of manganese, and caffeine also stimulates the thyroid).

When a baby is being born, or when a person is experiencing other stress, such as an infection, or when a person gets old, the best known thyroid hormone, thyroxine, is not changed to the more highly active form, T3 (triiodothyronine) in the normal way. In these emergency conditions, reduced oxygen consumption is a useful adaptation, since the blood is poorly oxygenated. Eating carbohydrate stimulates this conversion, so many additional calories of carbohydrate can be eaten without causing a weight gain (reviewed by C. Martin, 1978). Many people whose thyroid gland is suppressed by stress cannot respond to synthetic thyroxine, T4, since the same stress can block its conversion to T3. Natural thyroid, USP, is the most generally effective, but a non-prescription thyroid tablet is available at many health food stores.

Contrary to popular ideas about thyroid, the gland will resume its functioning after stopping the use of a supplement even if it has been suppressed, and sometimes taking thyroid will *increase* the gland's function to normal. Taking thyroid will sometimes help thin people gain weight, by improving protein metabolism, and it often helps people to sleep more soundly.

PROGESTERONE IN ORTHOMOLECULAR MEDICINE

In several ways, both progesterone and thyroid can be considered as primary regulatory hormones. Both of them regulate metabolism directly at the energetic and synthetic levels, both have a normalizing, anti-stress action on the pituitary, and each has a promoting action on the other. Both are blocked (or consumed) by stress, and promoted by light, and by good nutrition. Both oppose the effects of stress, and facilitate nutrition. Both *are* nutrients in cultures which eat the whole animal, including ovaries and thyroid.

Disregarding most of the information promoted by pharmaceutical companies, and the medical texts and journals which for thirty years have reflected the opinions of those companies (especially regarding the patented synthetic estrogens and glucocorticoids), we can trace a line of research and ideas on the sex hormones, from pioneers such as Loeb, Korenchevsky, and Selye, through a generation that continued to demonstrate the toxicity of estrogen, and the value of progesterone, including people like Lipschutz, Dalton and Soderwall. In my dissertation research under Soderwall, I had the opportunity to collect and assimilate data indicating an *increased* estrogen effect in aging animals, and recently, using radioimmunoassay for serum estrogen and progesterone, I have found a similar change in menopausal women, and Terry Parkening, who also studied under Soderwall, has used that technique to show that senescent infertility in mice is also associated with an increased ratio of estrogen to progesterone. My research showed that the probable mechanism by which estrogen excess causes infertility is through limiting the availability of oxygen. I showed that anti-estrogenic substances, such as progesterone or vitamin E, increased the oxygen tension in the uterus. This anti-oxygen effect of estrogen suggests a convergence of reproductive aging research with Warburg's theory that damaged respiration is the primary defect in cancer, and also with Selye's observation that estrogen's effect resembles the first, shock phase of the stress reaction.

Early research had also shown that estrogen diminishes hepatic glycogen (Brunelli, 1935), while progesterone increases both blood sugar and liver glycogen (Gaunt, et al., 1939). It is well known that hypoxia damages the fetal brain, **but probably less well known that hypoglycemia, either chronic or acute, can cause brain damage and retardation.** Hypoxia, by lowering metabolic efficiency, will cause hypoglycemia. Estrogen causes hypoxia at every imaginable site, from lung, through vascular fibrin and extracellular collagen and edema, to intracellular metabolism. Estrogen is also synergic with insulin, lowering blood sugar and promoting fat synthesis. Estrogen, and another common respiratory toxin, excessive unsaturated fats, have both been demonstrated to cause the birth of small-brained, retarded animals. Recent studies imply that about half of the children identified as hyperkinetic have experienced gestational stress. The most urgent need for progesterone therapy, I think, is in preventing a continuing epidemic of brain damage. Beyond that, many studies have found that the use of natural progesterone increases the child's IQ, typically by around 35 points (though there are claims of consistent 200 IQ's), and produces personalities that are more "independent, individualistic, self-assured, self-sufficient, and sensitive"

(J.M. Reinisch, *The Female Patient,* April, 1978, p. 87). Protection against hypoglycemia is probably the main mechanism — diabetic mothers often have precocious children, if they aren't damaged by drugs and irrational diets. Ten to fifteen grams per pregnancy, at increasing dosage, stopping a few days before expected delivery, seems to be the optimum amount, when there is some sign of excessive estrogen or expected toxemia, such as continuing menstruation in the first 2 or 3 months of pregnancy. The AMA department of drugs has specifically excluded progesterone from the sex hormones which are "now contraindicated in early pregnancy" ***(JAMA*** 239 (3) p.236).

Hypoglycemia (which can result from any respiratory defect) can produce malfunction of any tissue, but brain dysfunction and immune dysfunction are very common effects. Adamkiewics has shown that allergic reactions to a given substance will decrease from 100 percent to zero, when the blood glucose increases from, for example, 50 mg.% to 150 mg.% or more (also see Chernigovsky's book, Interoceptors). Progesterone (and thyroid) will help in most allergic diseases, including the autoimmune and "collagen diseases," because it helps to maintain blood sugar (promoting respiration and improving use of fat, sparing glucose) and also because it stabilizes lysosomes. This polar opposition of estrogen and progesterone also involves the polar antagonism of cyclic AMP and cyclic GMP, and to some extent a related antagonism of various prostaglandins (it has been suggested that this involves different populations of lysosomes, but I suspect it has to do with the superoxide dismutase enzyme system, and its inhibition or activation, since one of my assays to determine the action of estrogen turns out to be an inverse indicator of S.O.D. activity). Although progesterone and cortisone both raise blood sugar and stabilize lysosomes, their effect on the brain is very different: in large doses, progesterone is sedative and anesthetic, while cortisone is stimulating, and cortisone causes changes in the brain which resemble aging. The dopamine serotonin antagonism (e.g., in the control of prolactin secretion) can be modified by progesterone, thyroid, and other factors.

Pfeiffer has investigated the relationship of porphyria to certain forms of "schizophrenia," but I don't think he has mentioned that a good dose of glucose, or of an anti-estrogen hormone, such as testosterone or progesterone, will make the symptoms go away, just about as dramatically as Adamkiewics' glucose infusion will block inflammation or anaphylactic shock (incidentally, medical people just recently found that a large infusion of glucose was effective treatment in septic shock). Vitamin E, the old anti-estrogen, pro-fertility, pro-oxygen, anticlot nutrient, is now recognized as a factor in the control of porphyrin synthesis. Adaptively, it is logical for a lack of oxygen (as at high altitudes) to stimulate synthesis of the porphyrin ring, to use in respiratory systems, as hemoglobin or catalase. Other schizophrenias that Pfeiffer investigated involve disturbances in copper, zinc, and histamine, so it is interesting to note that these are powerfully regulated by estrogen, progesterone, and thyroid. Oxidation of epinephrine to adrenochrome has been seen in the uterus under the influence of estrogen, with copper as catalyst.

Other investigators have noticed abnormalities of pigmentation associated with psychoses or other nerve-related disease. Parkinson's disease, for example, involves degeneration of melanin-rich nerves, and melanin has now been identified as a "progesterone receptor," at least in some lower animals.

Most of the known biochemistry of lithium happens to overlap the actions of progesterone, e.g., aldosterone antagonism. However, while lithium has an anti-thyroid action, progesterone supports secretion of thyroxine, and apparently inhibits the formation of reverse T3, that chemical blocks the action of thyroid hormone. I have seen several women substitute progesterone for lithium, and several of these have then gone on to rely on nutrition and light.

While progesterone might seem to cure almost everything, we should be careful to use it only when the biochemical mechanism is fairly evident. A progesterone deficiency can be misdiagnosed, as (for example) epilepsy, Bright's disease, multiple sclerosis, or even estrogen deficiency (as in menopause). It can affect susceptibility to many conditions including herpes infections, dizziness, dysperception, varicose veins, mastitis, fibroma, and endometriosis. Cyclic edema, depression, and migraine are, in my experience, always stopped by progesterone. Sexual functions are often improved.

Progesterone is the precursor (following acetate and cholesterol) for all of the other steroid hormones, so it can be used in men. It (or its precursor, pregnenolone) has been used for prostatitis, arthritis, and infertility in men. Large amounts, though, would probably suppress LH, and lower testosterone synthesis, but a smaller amount (especially in old men) seems to increase sperm count and motility. In male and female athletes who become infertile, it would seem to be the appropriate therapy, generally in combination with thyroid.

Progesterone has been shown to be effective in many animal tumors, including pituitary tumors and other estrogen-induced tumors, and in human cervical and breast cancers. Since glucose metabolism is disturbed in cancer, it would seem reasonable to combine progesterone therapy with sufficient thyroid to maintain protein assimilation, and to provide a high protein diet to assure that the liver can excrete estrogen.

Even very intense emotional or perceptual symptoms typically disappear within 40 minutes when a dose of 300 mg. is given transdermally, dissolved in vitamin E or olive oil. Ovarian cysts, menopausal flushing, acne, sprains, and menstrual cramps can also be relieved with dramatic speed. In Addison's disease it can prevent some of the side effects of cortisone. Facial hair is often normalized in women. I have distributed about 25,000 doses of progesterone, and failure to use enough has been the most common problem. I always spend at least an hour with each person, learning about them and explaining relevant aspects of physiology and nutrition. I have each person read at least one book on the subject, such as the following:

K. Dalton, ***Premenstrual Syndrome and Progesterone Therapy*** (1978)
B. Barnes, ***Hypothyroidism, the Unsuspected Disease***
R. Peat, ***Mind and Tissue; Nutrition for Women;*** and my progesterone papers.

DOSAGE OF PROGESTERONE

Since progesterone is not known to have any side effects except for alteration of the menstrual cycle and production of euphoria (until doses of several grams per day are reached, at which point its anesthetic property begins to appear), the basic procedure should be to use it in sufficient quantity to make the symptoms disappear, and to time its use so that menstrual cycles are not disrupted. This normally means using it only between ovulation and menstruation unless symptoms are sufficiently serious that a missed period is not important. The basic idea of giving enough to stop the symptoms can be refined by some information on a few of the factors that condition the need for progesterone.

An excessive estrogen/progesterone ratio is more generally involved than either a simple excess of estrogen or a deficiency of progesterone, but even this ratio is conditioned by other factors, including age, diet, other steroids, thyroid, and other hormones. The relative estrogen excess seems to act by producing tissue hypoxia (as reported in my dissertation, University of Oregon, 1972), and this is the result of changes induced by estrogen in alveolar diffusion, peripheral vascular changes, and intracellular oxygen wastage.

Hypoxia in turn produces edema (as can be observed in the cornea when it is deprived of oxygen, as by a contact lens) and hypoglycemia (e.g., C. Martin: diminished ATP acts like insulin), because glycolysis must increase greatly for even a small deficiency of oxygen. Elevated blood lactic acid is one sign of tissue hypoxia. Edema, hypoglycemia, and lactic acidemia can also be produced by other "respiratory" defects, including hypothyroidism, in which the tissue does not use enough oxygen - the skin will be bluer (in thin places, such as around the eyes) when hypoxia, rather than low oxygen consumption, is involved. Low thyroid is one cause of excess estrogen; when both are involved, the color of the skin is neither red nor blue, but relatively bloodless white or yellow.

Symptoms in cycling women are most common around ovulation and in the premenstrual week, when the estrogen/progesterone ratio is normally highest. The early twenties and the late thirties and menopause are the ages when the ratio is most often disturbed - and these are also the ages when thyroid disorders are commonest in women.

Figure 1

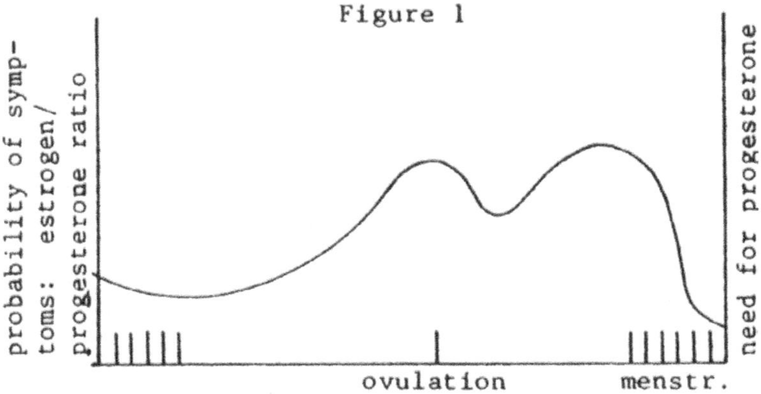

Besides a family tendency to have related symptoms, the individual who suffers from one aspect of the progesterone deficiency will tend to develop others at different times. With cyclic depressions or migraine headaches at age 22, there will possibly be breast disease and often there will be problems with pregnancy, and menopause may bring on a complete collapse.

Excess stress (by elevating estrogen and/or depleting progesterone, etc.) may bring on symptoms in someone who never had them. Spending a summer in Alaska, with an unusually long day, may relieve the symptoms of a chronic sufferer. Dark cloudy winters in England or the Pacific Northwest are powerful stressors, and cause lower progesterone in women and testosterone in men. Toxins, such as copper and lead, can produce similar symptoms. Porphyria and zinc deficiency are often caused by the hormone imbalance. A very common cause of an estrogen excess is a dietary protein deficiency - the liver simply cannot detoxify estrogen when it is undernourished (see Lipschutz references).

Figure 2

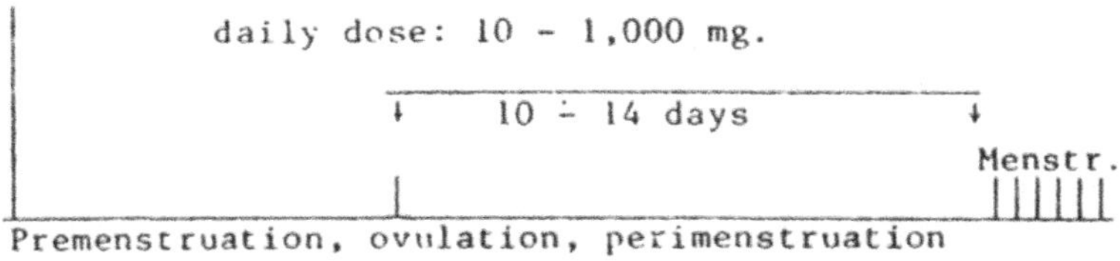

Figure 3

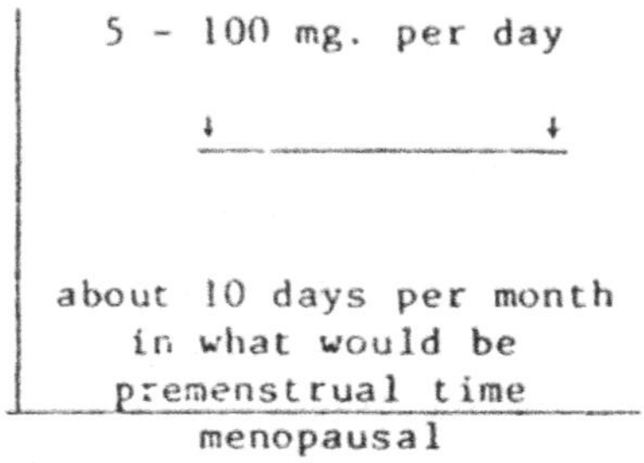

Figure 4

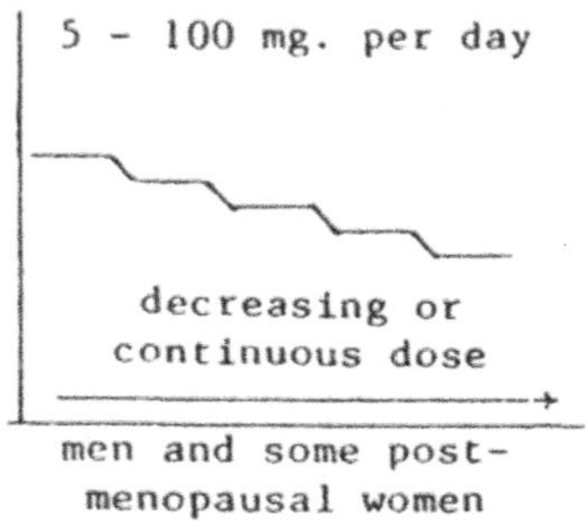

With a diet high in protein (e.g., 70-100 grams per day, including eggs) and vitamin A (liver once a week), I have found that the dose can be reduced each month. Using thyroid will usually reduce the amount of progesterone needed. Storage of progesterone apparently occurs in adipose tissue, so that one dose which is much bigger than needed will sometimes control the symptoms for several days.

Katharina Dalton, **Premenstrual Syndrome and Progesterone Therapy,** Year Book Medical Publishers, Inc., Chicago, 1977.

Alexander Lipschutz, **Steroid Hormones and Tumors,** Williams and Wilkens Company, Baltimore, 1950.

Raymond F. Peat, **Age Related Oxidative Changes In the Hamster Uterus,** University of Oregon thesis, Eugene, Oregon, 1972.

TRANSDERMAL PROGESTERONE FOR PREMENSTRUAL SYNDROME

For many years, Katharina Dalton' has studied the use of progesterone therapy for the premenstrual syndrome. A typical patient may require ten or more progesterone injections per month, more or less permanently. While this is feasible (at least in some countries) it is not comfortable or convenient, in some cases leads to serious reactions at the injection sites, and in the United States would be too expensive for general use. When the syndrome is disabling, even the burden of frequent and expensive injections is usually seen as a welcome alternative. However, a less expensive and more pleasant form of administration could make the therapy available to millions of women who are now disabled for one or more days each month. We are reporting here on what we believe to be a satisfactory alternative to the injection or implantation of progesterone, namely, a solution of progesterone and vegetable oil in a lotion or "cold cream" base for transdermal use.

After animal experiments revealed that progesterone in vegetable oil was absorbed effectively through the skin, in 1977 we began experiments with women who suffered from the premenstrual syndrome.

The effectiveness of the transdermal (absorption) route of administration varies with the individual, but compares favorably with injections in the amount assimilated. Thickness of skin or degree of circulation in the skin (these can be very abnormal in hypothyroidism, for example) and the amount of adipose tissue apparently make some difference in the rate of absorption and response. When a small daily dose (e.g., 5 or 10 mg.) is sufficient, this can be taken as about 250 mg. of a three percent cream rubbed into the throat, where it leaves no noticeable oiliness after a few minutes. For large doses, the appropriate amount can be applied to a larger area of skin after a hot bath, once or twice a day if necessary.

We have used transdermal progesterone therapy in two hundred women suffering from the full range of perimenstrual symptoms, including migraine, acne, depression, mastalgia, edema, and lethargy, and we found that nearly all of the women, applying the lotion themselves, are able to find the appropriate dosage for controlling their symptoms. Occasionally, thyroid therapy, weight reduction, or change in some aspect of lifestyle is necessary for complete relief from symptoms. We have learned that it is necessary to be very explicit in describing the amounts that can be used, while leaving it up to the patient to find the dose which controls her symptoms, because some women have an exaggerated idea of the power of a "hormone". We have learned, when some women said the progesterone had no effect, that they were applying it as sparingly as they would a rare perfume, just touching it to their wrists.

Another problem we have encountered is that a few women have trouble understanding how, if their edema is caused by "hormones", a "hormone" could relieve the edema. We have usually solved such problems by applying one dose (sometimes using a twenty-five percent solution) in the office, and waiting thirty or forty minutes to make sure that it was large enough to take effect. Once having felt sudden relief from this "cold cream", it is easier for the patient to understand how it should be used.

Unfortunately, many of the solvents which hold progesterone stably in a concentrated solution are highly allergenic. Injectable progesterone in oil could be used transdermally except for this problem. Progesterone can be removed from an injectable water suspension, and dissolved in warm olive or almond oil for transdermal use in patients who react to other solvents.

[1]Katharina Dalton, **The Premenstrual Syndrome and Progesterone Therapy,** Year Book Medical Publishers, Inc., Chicago, 1977.

TOPICAL PROGESTERONE FOR ACNE

In a previous study which found topical progesterone ineffective as therapy for acne, the investigators used ethanol as a solvent[1]. When water is added to a solution of progesterone and ethanol, the progesterone crystalizes out of solution, because water and ethanol have a fairly high mutual solubility and progesterone is practically insoluble in a water-ethanol mixture. When the progesterone-alcohol solution is applied to the skin, the alcohol takes up moisture from the skin, which is sufficient to cause the progesterone to be left undissolved on the surface. We have tried other solvents, including olive oil and vitamin E, which are stable in the presence of moisture, and we have had consistently positive results in twelve cases of acne associated with the menstrual cycle (usually appearing or getting worse around ovulation or just before menstruation) and in one of two teenage boys with chronic acne.

Because of the poor solubility, or instability of solution, of progesterone in natural oils of variable composition, we advised the patients to warm the solution in a hot water bath before every application. The solutions varied from one to ten percent progesterone (i.e., one to ten grams per 100 ml. of oil). Patients applied the oil to the affected skin once or twice a day. The amount of progesterone applied ranged from about 25 mg. per day to about 250 mg. per day.

The patients (except for one of the teenage boys, who reported no effect), consistently reported that use of progesterone at the first sign of a pimple stopped the development at that stage, prevented the expected outbreak, and within a few days resulted in a relatively clear skin. The improvement ranges from complete freedom from pimples in half of the group, to "improved, but still visible

---

[1] British Journal of Dermatology, Volume 99, Supplement 16, 9, July, 1978.

blemishes" in three women. Some of the solvents (sandalwood oil, vitamin E) caused an "allergic" skin irritation in two women, but switching to olive oil eliminated those reactions.

PROGESTERONE AND BODY TEMPERATURE

Women, more often than men, have "normal" body temperatures which are distinctly below normal, i.e., as low as 97 degrees, especially in the two weeks following menstruation. In men, giving progesterone doesn't cause an increase in body temperature, though it usually does in women. Progesterone is at its lowest in the two weeks between menstruating and ovulating. The fact that progesterone isn't "thermogenic" in men suggests that its activity relates to estrogen, which is its "antagonist." It is known that thyroid hormone increases heat production, and that estrogen is in many ways antagonistic to thyroxin. Therefore, it is not surprising that progesterone, by blocking estrogen's blockage of the thyroid hormone, should promote the effect of thyroxin and raise the temperature. The metabolism is shifted toward oxidation of fat, with the result that sugar is spared for the brain and kidneys and, in pregnancy, for the fetus.

Nutrition which supports the adrenals, ovaries, thyroid and liver can raise the body temperature toward normal, while reducing premenstrual symptoms and dysmenorrhea. Usually, vitamins A, E, pantothenic acid, and C will raise the temperature; sometimes other B complex vitamins are needed, as well as minerals such as iodine, manganese, zinc, and magnesium.

During stress, the temperature is often above normal, even when there are symptoms of progesterone deficiency. I have noticed that this is usually associated with enlarged lymph glands, as if the adrenal cortex had become inactive. In this state, adrenalin (and ACTH) would continue to be secreted, possibly at high levels, since the cortex normally makes anti-stress hormones to take over some of the resistance-promoting effects of adrenaline, if the stress lasts more than an hour or so. Adrenaline shrinks blood vessels in the skin (preventing heat loss) while stimulating metabolism and so might account for this fever of stress.

Sometimes progesterone seems to be chronically deficient (leading to slight — though possibly prolonged menstruation, or even amenorrhea), in women who exercise hard. Since progesterone can be converted into cortisone to handle stress, this could explain why well-trained athletes (who need lots of cortisone) so often miss periods. It seems to be a simple over-consumption of progesterone, which is probably a reasonable biological adaptation, preventing pregnancy during times of stress.

BREAST SORENESS, CYSTIC OVARIES

Women with benign breast diseases are likely to have abnormally low progesterone levels, while their estrogen stays relatively high (Mauvais-Jarvis, *Annales d'Endocrinologie* 37, 309-310, 1976). This same imbalance may also play a role in breast cancer (Sherman and Korenman, *Cancer* 33, 1506, 1974). Since progesterone is a chemical precursor of cortisol, prolonged stress would tend to lower the availability of progesterone, unless the adrenal glands are very well nourished. Vitamin A is required for progesterone synthesis, as well as for proper maturation of cells in membranes and glandular tissue. Pantothenic acid, niacin and vitamin C are commonly limiting factors in synthesis of adrenal hormones. (Synthetic "progestins" are likely to *cause,* rather than to prevent, breast cancer, and should never be used; natural progesterone needn't be injected, as some doctors believe, since it can be absorbed through the skin.) Cystic ovaries are often associated with sore breasts. Animal experiments (Janes; Leatham) show that lack of thyroid hormone can cause cystic ovaries. (See article on estrogen-thyroxin antagonism.)

2. STRESS

BLOOD SUGAR: SOME TECHNICAL BACKGROUND

Sugar can be used to produce energy with or without oxygen, but oxidative metabolism is about 15 times more efficient than the non-oxidative "glycolytic" or fermentative metabolism; higher organisms depend on this high efficiency oxidation for maintaining integration and normal functioning. If there is a small interference with respiration, the organism can adapt by increasing the rate of glycolysis, but there must be enough sugar to meet the demand. A response to stimulation is the production of more energy, with a proportional increase of oxygen and sugar consumption by the stimulated tissue; this produces more carbon dioxide, which enlarges the blood vessels in the area, providing more sugar and oxygen. If the irritation becomes destructive, efficiency is lost: oxygen is either consumed wastefully, causing blueness of the tissue (assuming circulation continues; blueness can also indicate bad circulation), or is not consumed, causing redness of the tissue. As more sugar is consumed in compensation, lactic acid also enlarges the blood vessels.

If the inflamed or exhausted tissue is small, the lactic acid can be consumed by other oxidizing tissues, sufficient sugar usually can be supplied, and repair occurs. But a large inflammation, or profound exhaustion, will lower the blood sugar systemically, and will deliver large amounts of lactic acid to the liver. The liver synthesizes glucose from the lactic acid, but at the expense of about 6 times more energy than is obtained from the inefficient metabolism — so that organismically, that tissue becomes 90 times less efficient than its original state. Besides this, an idle destruction of energy molecules (ATP or creatine phosphate) will increase the wastefulness even more.

When the organism detects the inflammation or other stress (possibly by sensing changes in blood sugar, lactic acid, or carbon dioxide, or all of them) its adrenal glands will secrete anti-stress hormones, including adrenalin and cortisone (assuming these glands are not exhausted or starved). Both adrenalin and cortisone can raise blood sugar to meet the increased need. Cortisone stimulates the conversion of protein to sugar, and since there are no "stored proteins" (other than small amounts circulating in the blood) this means that cortisone starts the conversion of the organism into fuel for the problem area. In acute emergencies, the lymphoid tissues will shrink first, which is all right, since they can be restored after the animal recovers, and their function — immunity — is partly a matter of a longer time scale, days to weeks. But if these tissues are chronically depleted by stress or malnutrition, infection is more likely to be fatal, as in old age or in poor populations. (The connection between infection, stress and sugar was illustrated recently by the discovery that infusing large amounts of glucose can relieve septic shock.)

Carbonated water can provide enough carbon dioxide (sometimes) to improve the delivery of blood (and glucose) to the brain. Low thyroid leads to low production of carbon dioxide and to wastage of glucose.

Various nutritional, hormonal, or toxic states interfere with respiration in different ways: for example, vitamin E deficiency, estrogen excess, toxic thyroid, and DNP (the formerly popular cancer-causing reducing drug) cause oxygen to be consumed without producing the normal amount of useful energy. Vitamin B2 or copper deficiency can prevent consumption of oxygen. Cancer (contrary to a tenacious establishment doctrine) involves a respiratory defect, and causes a tendency toward hypoglycemia which is often compensated by the conversion of protein to sugar, leading to the terminal wasting state (cachexia). (See Shapot and Blinov, *Cancer Research 34,* 1827-32, 1974.)

Vasodilation, edema, local heat and acidity are early responses to an irritant or energy defect; later, increased collagen production and capillary proliferation occur. Tumefaction and tissue death can result if the organism's resources aren't adequate.

Sugar wastage, leading to lactic acid production, can result from a vitamin B2 deficiency, and lactic acid appears to stimulate vascularization (Imre, 1964; *Exp. Eye Res.* 25, Supplement, 1977, P. 284). This would relate to the development of blood supply to cancers, and also to the blood-shot eyes and red noses and cheeks of alcoholics and others who are deficient in vitamin B2.

In general, stress should be met first by correcting the defect, which may be environmental or nutritional. Increased nutritional needs usually include protein and fat; acute hypoglycemia may require a large amount of sugar, and this suggests that the adrenals may be depleted, in which case pantothenic acid, vitamin C, vitamin A, magnesium and potassium should be provided in addition to other nutrients.

Sometimes, sugar has to be eliminated permanently to control hypoglycemia. Some people have to eat a snack (e.g., a small slice of cheese) every hour, but this can often be overcome if the liver is able to recuperate.

Pantothenic acid is needed by the liver to destroy insulin (insulinase), so hyperinsulinism, causing hypoglycemia, can sometimes be remedied with this nutrient.

STRESS AND SPECIAL NUTRITIONAL REQUIREMENTS

According to Hans Selye, activation or injury of tissue is the beginning of stress. The more cells involved, the greater is the stress. An injury to a leg connected only by blood vessels produces a stress reaction in the animal, so the signal of stress can be transmitted in the blood, though the nerves are normally also involved. Adenine nucleotides have been suspected as a cause of shock (because they are vasodilators, as are many other products of stress, including phosphate), but other possibilities are histamine, various polyamines, and low blood sugar.

Selye divides stress into three phases: alarm, resistance (or adaptation), and exhaustion. Three tissues are usually the first to show effects: thymolymphatic tissue shrinks, gastrointestinal tissue becomes inflamed and bleeds, and the adrenal cortex becomes enlarged.

Selye classifies steroids into anti- and pro-inflammatory. Inflammation is a relatively non-specific, and hopefully local, reaction, serving to isolate the problem if it is a toxin or infection. Cortisol is a typical anti-inflammatory hormone; DOC (deoxycorticosterone) is considered by Selye to be a natural pro-inflammatory steroid, but other endocrinologists point out that it is normally present only in very small amounts, as a precursor of aldosterone (which helps retain sodium in stress — sodium probably helps activate the glycolytic pathway, speeding the use of sugar). Some of Selye's stress experiments involved giving a large dose of sodium, presumably increasing the amount of DOC in the tissues, and intensifying stress symptoms.

Injury and exertion have in common the need for more fuel. I think the blood sugar level is therefore useful at least for understanding stress, even if other substances are involved in the "signaling" or coordinating process. From my own experience, I am inclined to believe that blood sugar is an important integrating factor, and that the organism can probably sense small or rapid fluctuations that would be very hard to detect by the usual laboratory procedures. For example, males in particular are known to secrete adrenaline under the stress of having blood drawn, and this tends to raise the concentration of blood sugar. Even when extremely large and prolonged variations in blood sugar are found, the concept of "normal range" allows most physicians to dismiss them as being insignificant — even when the patient develops classical symptoms of hypoglycemia: if the patient faints or has convulsions when his blood sugar falls 50 mg.%, the physician is likely to note the "psychosomatic reaction" or the "coincidental epilepsy," since a "normal variation" in blood sugar concentration supposedly couldn't be responsible. More physicians are now recognizing that the rate of fall can be as important as the absolute level.

Hans Selye sometimes used an injected metal, such as iron salts, to experimentally sensitize animals to stress, making it easier to produce arthritis. He found that vitamin E could offset this effect of iron.

SUGAR AND THE PANCREAS

Ordinary refined cane or beet sugar is sucrose, a "double sugar" or disaccharide. (Some of this chemical terminology is useful for understanding food labels.) The two units making up sucrose are glucose and fructose. These are monosaccharides, and since they contain six carbon atoms, they can also be called hexoses. Glucose is classed as an “aldose" because it contains an aldehyde group: by just shifting the position of two hydrogen atoms onto this aldehyde group, glucose turns into fructose (a keto sugar or ketose").

Carbohydrates are usually split into monosaccharides before being absorbed. They are carried to the liver, where glucose can be used to replenish the storage form **of** carbohydrate, glycogen. If there is more glucose than the liver can store, it reaches the pancreas where it stimulates the release of insulin, which disposes of the sugar by stimulating synthesis of fat and glycogen. The insulin is only slowly degraded, so it will go on lowering blood sugar if sugar isn't being absorbed continuously from the gut. If blood sugar gets too low, an alarm reaction will produce adrenalin to restore blood sugar, with the result that the person may feel anxious.

Insulin should be about 30% destroyed by the liver each time the blood circulates to the liver, but a pantothenic acid deficiency will prevent this regulation. Low thyroid also interferes with liver function limiting the storage and release of glycogen.

Fructose doesn't stimulate the pancreas as glucose does. It is gradually converted into glucose. In people with high blood lipids, however, it is utilized by liver and fat tissues several times faster than it is in normal people: it is as if the cellular "doors" were already open in these people, maybe as a result of high insulin levels, and the cells accept fructose more rapidly than normal. This doesn't imply that fructose is to be avoided as rigidly as is glucose, since I don't think there is any evidence that it initiates any problem. Grapes are rich in glucose; other fruits have varying quantities of fructose: honey contains some fructose. Jerusalem artichokes that have been kept in storage are a very good source of fructose. Onions are another source. I suspect that even glucose wouldn't be so hard on the body if it were always taken with potassium and other nutrients involved in its metabolism.

Potassium is necessary for utilization of sugar, and should probably always be tried as a supplement in the diabetic diet, especially since fruits, an important source of potassium, may be avoided because of their sugar. Some B vitamins (B1 and B2 and probably niacin) are said to have similar effects on the utilization of sugar. Some forms of diabetes involve normal or high levels of insulin, others, a lack of insulin; both have been found to respond to nutrition, but especially the high insulin form. The pancreas can be damaged by prolonged malnutrition, so that the inability to produce insulin may be permanent. Magnesium and vitamin B6 deficiencies are known to be involved in damage to the pancreas. Insulin itself is only part of the "insulin-like" system *(Adv in Metabol Disorders 7,* p.26, 1974); proper treatment requires a proper study of all factors. I know of children who have been put immediately on insulin for life, after one urine test showed glucose, even though the test followed a stressful infection. Stress can cause sugar to appear in the urine, as can many other conditions, and this does not call for insulin treatment.

EMOTIONAL PROBLEMS

Just before menstruation begins, and just after giving birth, the level of estrogen in the body can be high, and out of proportion to other hormones. Tension, anxiety, depression, being too easily upset emotionally, and even having hallucinations can result from this hormone imbalance. Excess estrogen causes the body to accumulate copper, and copper poisoning itself (often caused by water that is contaminated, for example by plumbing, a hot water heater, or utensils) is known to cause symptoms of schizophrenia. Menopause is another time of frequent emotional upsets, for many women. A type of psychosis sometimes occurs at menopause. Since it is easier to test for excess copper than for excess estrogen, it might be worthwhile to have this test done when there are emotional problems during menopause, around menstruation, or in the first few weeks after giving birth. Tension resulting from too much copper or estrogen can be relieved nutritionally. Usually a zinc supplement is necessary — about 20 mg. a day; about 30 mg. of vitamin B6 has been recommended for this problem, but the amount varies with the individual. The other B vitamins, and vitamins E and A should also be used. Sometimes as much as 500 mg. of niacin can be required to stop a "hysterical" feeling. The mildly sedative action of magnesium can also have a dramatic effect. One half to one gram of magnesium is enough if it is taken in a highly soluble (and assimilable) form such as magnesium chloride. Since low blood sugar is often a factor in anxiety or depression, adequate protein and calories must be eaten regularly. Biotin (1-2 mg.) can stop some depressions. Fruit is very useful in maintaining blood sugar since it provides sugar with potassium which helps to avoid an insulin reaction.

PEOPLE DIAGNOSED AS "PSYCHOTIC"

Women are increasingly being diagnosed as "manic-depressive," though this used to be thought of as mainly a man's disease. I think the new popularity of lithium "therapy" has contributed to this diagnostic trend. Even if the problem is what had previously been described as "premenstrual depression," lithium therapy does work, though some patients complain of tremor, dullness, and clumsiness.

Several of the known biochemical effects of lithium are similar to those of progesterone, including antagonism to aldosterone, modification of serotonin metabolism, elevation of nerve thresholds, and facilitated disposition of ammonia. (Other psycho-active chemicals which have some overlap with progesterone are DOPA, bromocriptine, and physostigmine.)

One type of "schizophrenia," and the very common symptom of "agoraphobia" or reclusiveness, are associated with high levels of porphyrins and pyrroles. Fasting, liver damage, and increased estrogen levels can raise the concentrations of certain of these substances; they seem to promote urinary loss of zinc and vitamin B6. Estrogen promotes copper (and iron, and calcium) retention, and copper tends to displace zinc. The high levels of copper, iron and lead which are found in many people with mental problems may be secondary to a hormone disturbance. Thyroid gland or progesterone, or both, can produce a complete disappearance of mental symptoms when those symptoms result from any biochemical imbalance that can be rectified hormonally, because these two substances have very generalized regulatory functions. I feel that any "diagnosis" (naming in Latin) of a "functional mental disturbance" is at best irrelevant, and may be very destructive. People with diagnoses of "schizophrenia," "epilepsy," "manic-depressive psychosis," "Parkinsonism," "myasthenia gravis," "involutional psychosis," "neuritis," "sclerosis," etc., have reported that they felt normal or improved after taking progesterone, often within 40 minutes. Magnesium, as epsom salts or magnesium chloride or carbonate, can relieve some cases of irritability and tension, even when something else, such as hypothyroidism, is the basic cause.

Many symptoms have been blamed on cerebral edema, which might result from too much estrogen. However, the speed with which some symptoms disappear suggest other possible explanations. Just as veins in the forehead shrink immediately if a ***large*** amount of sugar is taken for a migraine, I have seen veins (back of hand) disappear with progesterone treatment, just when a suicidal depression is lifting. This suggests that there may be a "migraine" condition in the blood vessels of the limbic system of the brain, but there are also very rapid shifts in brain chemistry.

Light and smell are known to affect hormone production. A musky material (Le Magnen's "exaltolide," probably includes androstenol) is probably a social regulator of hormones — perfume containing musk might affect the woman who wears it. Bright lights for 18 hours per day can correct some hormone-mood problems.

Canker sores, herpes infections, and bleeding gums, if associated with mental symptoms, suggest a thyroid and/or progesterone deficiency.

CANCER PRODUCES STRESS

Cancer overstimulates the anti-stress adrenocortical hormones, and usually produces extreme wasting from mobilization of fat and protein; blood sugar and glycogen storage are disturbed. During or after cancer treatment the "hypoglycemia" diet seems desirable: frequent small feedings, liver (or similar nutrients), magnesium, potassium. Vitamins A, E, C, and pantothenic acid are particularly important in stress, but all nutrients are necessary.

In an article on inflammation, the Encyclopedia Britannica makes this comment which is extremely interesting in connection with the fact that cancer involves a failure of the immune reaction:

> Severe starvation or...deficiency of protein may restrict antibody formation. Hormones of the adrenal cortex in sufficient amounts depress formation of certain types of antibody. The adrenal cortex secretions are capable of altering the inflammatory reaction in several ways: excessive amounts of the hydrocortisone type of secretion reduce the quantity of exudate formed and the amount of fibrous tissue and capillary proliferation.

About 1950, prisoners were experimentally injected with cancer cells; those who already had cancer developed tumors where cells were injected; healthy patients apparently never developed cancer, though a reasonable follow-up wasn't done. Cortisone treatment is known to speed growth and spreading of injected cancer cells. Cancer patients are typically unable to even produce a normal inflammation, as if they are powerfully dosed with the anti-stress cortisone-type hormones. The failure of the immune system, which can normally wipe out cancer cells as they develop, seems to be an essential feature of cancer, and as quoted above, adrenocortical hormones can suppress antibody formation; the conversion of body protein to sugar (an effect of these hormones) causes shrinking of the thymus gland, which is essential for healthy immune reactions. Although there may be other things involved in the immune suppression, part of it appears to be this drain on the body's protein, which can be alleviated nutritionally. Dr. W. D. Kelly *(One answer to cancer)* describes an interesting test for cancer based on this problem in protein metabolism. A drop of blood squeezed from a puncture in the finger should stand up in a spherical drop, but when a person is developing cancer, it spreads instead of rounding up. (See the section on edema) Stress apparently increases a person's need for all nutrients including calories and protein. The vitamins most commonly used for resisting stress are A, C, E, and pantothenic acid. The minerals magnesium, calcium, potassium and zinc can help in the first stages of stress, and sodium supplements may be needed in the last extreme stage of stress when the adrenals have been exhausted.

ARTHRITIS AND STRESS

Dr. E. C. Barton-Wright and Dr. **W.** A. Elliot have found pantothenic acid (at least 25 to 50 milligrams per day) useful in arthritis. Arthritis is commonly a result of stress; stress increases the need for that vitamin and also for other nutrients including vitamins A and C. Arthritis often follows surgery. Sometimes surgery can bring on chronic allergic problems (hay fever, gas, fatigue, etc.) but it can also apparently weaken the immune system so badly that old allergies disappear after an operation.

Stress inhibits the thyroid, and can lower progesterone (and/or testosterone) while raising estrogen. Recent work by Siiteri and his group shows a hormonal involvement in various "autoimmune" diseases. Females are much more susceptible to these sicknesses than are males. Systemic lupus erythematosus and rheumatoid arthritis are common.

Vitamin A offsets a protein deficiency, and a protein deficiency can damage immunity.

Any activity, if planned and completed according to plan without interruption, can reduce stress. Enforced inactivity, and inability to achieve what was intended, are powerful stressors. The adrenal hormones and mineral metabolism are disturbed in stress, whether the cause is a disorganized style of life, or the injury of surgery. The diet should include about 90 grams of protein (in frequent feedings), eggs as a source of sulfur (needed to synthesize joint lubricants, for example), and should keep the ratio of magnesium to calcium high (as with vegetables, bran, fruit), and the phosphate intake low (this would include using green leaves in place of some meat, as well as using cheese). Vitamins C, E, and pantothenic acid are needed in especially large amount in stress. Vitamins A and B2 are also essential for production of the anti-stress hormones. Inositol is known to protect biological materials from many kinds of damage, and might have this effect in arthritis, but I don't know of any research in this particular application.

Iron salts, and other heavy metals, have been shown by Hans Selye to produce arthritis, possibly by their ability to destroy vitamins E and C.

Copper is a "specific" oxidant for vitamin C. It is associated with many inflammatory diseases, and should probably be better investigated in "degenerative" diseases, including arthritis and glaucoma.

Pantothenic acid in very large doses was recently found to protect against stress even when an animal's adrenals were removed. Since the nutrient is needed to destroy insulin, I think part of its anti-stress effect comes from minimizing hypoglycemia, and so reducing the amount of cortisone needed.

On the cellular level, stress lowers the energy charge. Systemically, stress inhibits oxidative metabolism. Both of these observations indicate that the "basic" anti-stress hormone would be thyroid. Hypothyroidism often involves arthritis — sometimes the tiny bones of the ear which transmit sound are affected. Ringing of the ears and deafness for high sounds are common in hypothyroidism

M. Kirchgassner and H.L. Mueller, The effect of varying the protein diet on the trace elements content of early-weaned piglets." *Landwirtsch Forsch 27* (314), p. 358-364, 1974: "copper/dry body matter clearly fell when the protein supply was increased." (And zinc rose.)

CORTISONE

About 25 years ago cortisone was found to increase the metastatic spread of cancer. Since it raises blood sugar by dissolving protein from the tissues, the immune system and muscles are damaged. When the muscle mass is diminished, loss of fat becomes more difficult. Vitamin A can apparently help offset immunosuppression by cortisone. Use of cortisone can result in puffiness and water retention. It is a way of exaggerating the body's normal hormone response to stress, and may be justified if the adrenal glands are damaged. Pantothenic acid and vitamins C and A can help restore the glands' natural activity.

Vitamin B2 deficiency is also known to affect the adrenal glands, and has been suspected of contributing to the development of Addison's disease.

Vitamin A offsets a protein deficiency, and a protein deficiency can damage immunity.

Cortisone causes the liver to produce estrogen.

PREGNENOLONE

Pregnenolone is the first steroid produced from cholesterol, under the influence of thyroid and vitamin A. Large amounts are produced in the brain, by certain glial cells that are one of our essential anti-stress systems. The need for producing pregnenolone is associated with a sense of being under stress, and taking a supplement of pregnenolone causes many fatigued, stressed people to have a renewed sense of ability to meet challenges. Ordinarily, thyroid hormone supplementation has the same effect by promoting the conversion of cholesterol to pregnenolone, but when there isn't enough cholesterol, or when the mitochondria have accumulated damage (such as might be produced by tissue accumulation of iron, displacing copper), pregnenolone itself seems to be needed. For many years, I have felt that the skin might be one of our most important endocrine organs, and it has been demonstrated that it is able metabolize various steroids. I suspect that pregnenolone is as important to the skin as it is to the brain. Several years ago, I noticed that my facial skin, that had gradually seemed to loosen with aging, suddenly contracted back to a snugger, more elastic fit shortly after I started taking a small amount of pregnenolone. Since then, I have seen the same thing happen in other people; one man said it was like an overnight face lift, when he took a large amount, that also had a profound effect on his mood. A few years ago, the fiber cells, which are a major component of the skin, were found to contain the same contractile materials that muscles have. I think pregnenolone allows these cells to contract, restoring firmness to slack skin. Pregnenolone can quickly cause other very rapid "anatomical" changes, though, that seem to have more to do with eliminating edema, than with contraction of cells, such as causing protruding eyes (in Graves' disease) to recede, or causing joint cartilage to function normally and painlessly, or causing lungs to oxygenate the blood efficiently in people with emphysema. The chart in the appendix on page 153 shows some of the factors involved in the formation of pregnenolone.

3. AGING

Some people who are supposed to be "experts" quite crazily claim that what you eat has nothing to do with how fast you age. Experiments with animals, observations of other cultures, and even some experiments with humans have shown clearly that nutrition can have a profound effect on the body changes which are called aging. In the three regions where a very high proportion of the population lives to be more that 100, the average daily calorie intake is only about 1500, which is considered "inadequate" by most nutritionists. Animals which are kept on a low calorie diet live much longer than those that are fed more, so we can assume that the low calorie diet contributes to the long life of those three groups. However, other similarities have been found in the diets in those three regions. Their food is fresh, they use a lot of animal fat (e.g., milk and cheese), they regularly eat greens, and some of them tend to drink quite a bit of alcohol, though in unrefined forms such as wine.

All of the essential nutrients are needed constantly to prevent deterioration of the body. At different times, nutrients such as vitamin C, pantothenic acid, or vitamin E, have been identified as methods to prevent premature aging. In our culture, many people do have severe deficiencies of those nutrients, but any dietary deficiency can cause degenerative changes. I have experimentally reversed a variety of degenerative changes with special nutrition, but the problem always exists within a particular person's physiology, and can't necessarily be solved by a standardized diet. You have to learn to know what your body needs at a particular time. This will be made easier if your basic diet is roughly like that described above — moderately low calorie intake, fairly high protein intake, with high quality proteins such as eggs, milk, and leaves, and with fresh fruit or vegetables every day.

Study of many different species, including humans, shows that aging is slower in individuals that have a larger brain in relation to body size. Brain size is strongly influenced both by prenatal nutrition and by nutrition in early childhood. The first year and a half is extremely important for the development of intelligence, since brain cells are still becoming more numerous up to that age, but growth and development of the brain can still be stunted by poor nutrition later. Progesterone is an important factor in brain development: estrogen inhibits brain development. Unsaturated fats also inhibit brain development if used in excess, and recent studies show that they also increase visible aging of the skin.

MENOPAUSAL FLUSHING

I have talked to several women in their 20s who complained of sensations of heat around their heads, night sweats, sudden flushing, and other symptoms that are associated with the menopause. Katharina Dalton has found that premenstrual symptoms, which result from a relative estrogen surplus and a progesterone deficiency, often continue during the menopause. Siiteri and his group have discovered that one of the steroids (androstenedione, usually associated with the male hormones) is converted to a form of estrogen at an increasing rate as a person gets older, at all ages they studied, from 20 to 80, in both men and women. Strickler found that only 10% of his patients with menopausal symptoms such as flushing, could feel and benefit from estrogen when it was alternated with a placebo. These studies, and a few dozen others, have convinced me that the symptoms of menopause result mainly from a progesterone deficiency, relative to the estrogens. The 10% who really feel better from estrogen *possibly* have an estrogen deficiency, but this has not been determined, and several other things could account for the "lift" they feel for example, a *healthy* thyroid gland will respond to elevated estrogen with an increased output of thyroxin, which at least would make the person feel different, and might raise blood sugar, increase alertness, etc.

In 1979 menopausal flushing was found to be associated with an elevation of the pituitary hormone, LH. A lack of progesterone is known to cause a rise in LH.

Digitalis and progesterone have very similar effects on the heart (Szent-Gyorgyi, *Muscle Contraction).* Digitalis is able to raise blood pressure and increase urine production, apparently by increasing the tone of the arterioles (Abram, 1910). If progesterone's effect on muscle includes such an effect on arterioles, then the "puzzle" of menopausal — and premenopausal — flushing is no puzzle, but is merely one symptom of a progesterone deficiency relative to estrogen. Progesterone does have a diuretic effect, but this has been attributed to an antagonism to aldosterone, rather than to an effect on arterioles.

Besides the nutrients needed to regulate the estrogen level (protein and B vitamins) and nutrients needed by the thyroid (e.g., iodine, manganese, and cobalt), special attention should be given to the anti-stress vitamins which are involved in progesterone synthesis (vitamin A, pantothenic acid, vitamin C, vitamin E) and to the nutrients that are known to be "wasted" by excess estrogen: folic acid, zinc, and vitamin B6, particularly. Vitamin B6 is needed to synthesize materials that regulate blood vessel tone and that act as brain modulators, governing sleep, emotions, alertness, etc. Memory of dreams is said to be promoted by adequate B6 (Pfeiffer, 1975). White marks on the fingernails, especially of the right hand, are suggestive of a zinc deficiency. Brittle fingernails are likely to result from too much estrogen. or inhibited thyroid function; vitamin A and eggs are useful, but calcium and gelatin are not. Magnesium carbonate is very useful for stabilizing nerves and muscles while raising the energy level: one gram a day of magnesium is a reasonable amount, but many tablets now contain only 15 to 50 mgs.

Dalton, K., *The Premenstrual Syndrome,* C. Thomas. Springfield, Ill., & London, 1964.

Hemsell, et al., Plasma precursors of estrogen. II. Correlation of the extent and conversion of plasma androstenedione to estrone with age, *J. Clin. Endocrinol. Metab.* 38, p. 476, 1974.

Grodin, et al., Source of estrogen production in postmenopausal women, *J. Clin. Endocrinol Metab* 36. p. 207, 1973.

Strickler, *Contemporary Ob /Gyn,* August, 1976.

Mulley and Mitchell, *Lancet,* June 26, 1976, p. 1397, "Is estrogen therapy justified in menopausal flushing?"

C.C. Pfeiffer, *Mental and Elemental Nutrients,* Keats Publ. Co., 1975.

SIMILARITY OF MENOPAUSE AND CUSHING'S SYNDROME

Excess estrogen is known to cause hypertrophy of the adrenal cortex. Since estrogen stimulates insulin release and lowers blood sugar, the hypertrophy may be to compensate by raising blood sugar.

The distribution of fat is similar in aging and in Cushing's syndrome. Vitamin E is known to shift enzyme activities in a way that would offset this distribution, and this might occur in cases caused by hormone disturbances other than mere aging.

The fall of spermine which occurs in senility, in estrogen excess, and in hypoglycemia should also be investigated in Cushing's syndrome.

The changes in endometrium, and the "castrate" type of vaginal epithelium are similar in both states. (Is the influence of contraceptive pills on vaginal epithelium what causes pain in intercourse?)

Osteoporosis and diabetes are frequently part of Cushing's syndrome, and are also more common after the menopause. Cortisone therapy (even when used on the skin) can cause mineral loss — recently an 8 year old girl who had stopped growing was found to have osteoporosis resulting from use of a cortisone ointment. Thyroxine elevates magnesium levels in the tissue and is known to promote bone regeneration and mineralization. Estrogen's antagonism to thyroxin is so general that we could suspect that it would also inhibit healthy mineralization. Estrogen has long been used during and after the menopause for its supposed ability to prevent osteoporosis, but this is now known to be incorrect: any beneficial effect it has on osteoporosis is only temporary (C. Martin, *Textbook of Endocrine Physiology,* 1976).

In animal experiments, it has been found that cortisone can produce diabetes, apparently by damaging the pancreas, and it has been suspected that chronic stress (which can be brought on by low blood sugar) can be a factor in producing diabetes.

Aging, stress, menopause, Cushing's syndrome, and the premenstrual syndrome all overlap so much that each state can probably give us some insight into the others. An elevated estrogen/progesterone ratio is likely to be a common feature.

CHOLESTEROL

A recent newspaper article about a former Oregon politician says He was in excellent physical condition." "So for all these years, he hasn't smoked, he's kept his weight down to his normal 165 pounds. He has cut down on eating fatty foods and has watched his diet carefully." "I was in good shape," he said in his hospital room after being treated for the nearly fatal heart attack he had while jogging. I quote this because it shows how taking certain stylish "precautions" can give a person a false sense of security. Since a healthy liver will produce cholesterol to make up for what is lacking in the diet, avoiding high cholesterol foods won't necessarily lower blood cholesterol. In an article called "Fat has less cholesterol than lean," Raymond Reiser of Texas A & M University points out that 100 grams of a chicken drumstick has 91 mg. of cholesterol, while pork has only about 60 mg. per 100 grams. "On the calorie basis," he says, the cholesterol content of lean cuts "is about 4 to 6.6 times as high" as that of fat.

Vitamin C is now known to lower blood cholesterol. Eggs are rich in cholesterol, but they also contain lecithin, which appears to make the cholesterol useful, or at least less harmful. Niacin and vitamin E also help to regulate cholesterol. High insulin levels, caused by eating sugar, seem to be important in allowing cholesterol to damage the blood vessels. Cholesterol is used in the production of many hormones, including sex and anti-stress hormones.

High cholesterol usually indicates low thyroid function. When thyroid is low, cholesterol isn't converted efficiently into progesterone. The real cause of heart attacks seems to be hypothyroidism and its effects, including loss of magnesium. Stressful exercise can aggravate hypothyroidism.

AGING SKIN

Although estrogen is known to advance the aging of collagen in all tissues that have been studied, including skin, it has been promoted as a "youth drug." The beef industry uses it because it makes cows swell up with fat and water, to increase profits: it is no longer legal to soak meat — except ham — in water before weighing it for sale. Women, like cows, will puff up with water and fat under the influence of estrogen, and wrinkles will naturally be smoothed out, but the skin itself is actually losing its elasticity faster when estrogen is used. Testosterone and progesterone both have direct anti-estrogen activity. Testosterone lotion was tested on one armpit of an old woman. Her tissue had atrophied so that there was no hair, the sweat glands didn't function, and the skin was thin and wrinkled. After several weeks of daily use of the lotion, hair and sweat glands had returned to normal, and the skin was thicker, firmer, and smoother (photographs were published). Her other armpit remained as before. Progesterone has been found to reverse the chemical changes which occur in collagen with aging. In pregnancy, progesterone is probably responsible for the formation of relaxin, a hormone which makes the fibrous tissues become very stretchy, so the birth canal can open without damage. Some women notice that joints become very limber for a few days every month, suggesting that relaxin can be formed even when the woman is not pregnant.

Some of the changes of aging probably relate to "autoimmune" reactions, in which the body attacks itself; both testosterone and progesterone normalize the immune system, suppressing auto-immune problems. There are several dietary practices which will promote the formation of progesterone, but the most effective is to use liver once a week, to use eggs daily, and to avoid foods which inhibit the thyroid, such as raw cabbage and broccoli. Butter contains some progesterone. Young women might grow moustaches if they used testosterone cream on their skin very often (one day a month, at ovulation, women normally produce considerable testosterone) but natural progesterone lotion could be used safely for its effect on collagen. Progesterone has also been used to eliminate excess facial hair (photographs of this effect of progestins have been published in the *J. of Steroid Biochemistry).*

Synthetic hormones are certain to have side effects.

ESTROGEN AND OSTEOPOROSIS, ETC.

Estrogen has been promoted (on grounds that are at best dubious) as a therapy for menopause, for aging skin, for heart disease, for cancer, for premenstrual syndrome, for endometriosis, for preventing miscarriages, for nervousness and depression, for abnormal bleeding, and for osteoporosis. From Sept. 21, 1977, drug companies are required to give doctors and druggists brochures with estrogen, warning of the risk of cancer, and advising that estrogen not be given for nervousness, depression, or for "restoring youthfulness" during menopause, because it is ineffective for those purposes (UPI, July 20-21, 1977). However, they failed to mention studies which had already reported that estrogen causes, rather than cures, heart attacks. It causes a magnesium deficiency, which promotes clotting (Seelig and Heggtveit. *Amer. J. Clin. Nutr. 27,* pp. 59-79, 1974). The magnesium deficiency also promotes abnormal fat metabolism, contributing to heart disease. Even before estrogen was chemically identified, it was known to promote breast cancer; in the 1930s it was shown to cause tissue aging, fibroid tumors, various cancers, premenstrual syndrome and menstrual abnormalities, and to induce abortions. Nevertheless, from 1947 to 1964 a synthetic estrogen, DES, already demonstrated to be highly toxic, was prescribed to millions of women to *prevent* miscarriages. When women succeeded in having babies in spite of this mistreatment, it typically caused girl babies to later develop vaginal cancer, and many of the boy babies grew up to be sterile. By the early 1960s it was apparent that birth control drugs had a bigger market than drugs for the miscarriage trade, so DES was switched over to use in birth control pills, and is still widely used as a morning after pill." Since estrogen was known to cause obesity and edema, it occurred to someone that there would be a really big market for DES in the meat industry: chickens, turkeys and cows with edema weigh more, and gross fatness not only increases the animals' weight, it also fills out the skin so the animal looks smooth and plump. (The same effect of plumpness has been sold to women as "young skin," even though estrogen actually causes aging of the connective tissue in skin.) Meat graders have said that DES lowers the quality of the meat (apart from the residue toxicity), but the increased weight makes it a profitable practice.

By 1950, any normally perceptive person was aware that physicians were doing things exactly backwards in many cases. This was not the result of a new homeopathic philosophy, or the "hair of the dog that bit you" theory. It was the result of drug companies' having their patented products, and knowing how to use the medical establishment for their own purposes, without regard to science. Their huge profits allowed them to spend several thousand dollars each year on each physician, sometimes including gifts of color television sets and free vacations, and discounts on things for the doctors' own use. Probably the most terrible use of their wealth was the gradual reversal of scientific opinion, achieved through grants to scientists who got the results they wanted, and cancellation of grants when the results went the wrong way, and through financial support for professional meetings and publications, and through influence on the editorial policies of medical journals by the threatened withholding of advertising.

Probably the last, strongest argument for the widespread use of estrogen is that it supposedly delays the development of osteoporosis. The absence of osteoporosis in old women in many other countries is never discussed in the professional meetings on osteoporosis subsidized by the drug companies. Constance Martin, in her ***Textbook of Endocrine Physiology,*** (1976), says that **"estrogens are not useful if administered over long periods of time...."** M.R. Urist (in ***Biochem. and Physiol. of Bone, vol.2,*** G.H. Bourne, 1972 ed.) says that estrogen doesn't restore bone mass “to a degree demonstrable by roentgenography," that excessive growth hormone "may aggravate" the disorder, and that estrogen stimulates the release of growth hormone. The argument for using estrogen to cure or prevent osteoporosis is based on the fact that estrogen causes diminished urinary excretion of calcium. A vitamin E deficiency (and estrogen is known to increase the need for vitamin E) causes calcium to be retained by muscles. Any toxin, in fact, causes calcium retention in the soft tissues —

for example, when the heart is deprived of oxygen, it absorbs calcium. Since no skeletal improvement can be demonstrated by x-rays, I suspect that the improved calcium retention is merely a toxic effect of estrogen. A proper control in this sort of experiment would be to compare the effect of toxins such as iodoacetate and cyanide, with the effect of estrogen.

BLOOD PRESSURE - VITAMIN E AND OTHER NUTRIENTS

The kidneys produce a material which raises blood pressure, and the production of this chemical is increased when the supply of oxygen is not adequate. Other tissues probably produce similar chemicals. Normally, as soon as the blood pressure is increased, circulation is improved so that an adequate amount of oxygen is delivered to the tissues. However, there are many processes that can waste oxygen, and some of these tend to increase gradually with age, so that the blood pressure rises steadily over the years.

General tissue damage, malnutrition, and hormone imbalance can all produce conditions in which oxygen is consumed without producing a normal amount of energy. Also, a failure of the small blood vessels to open properly can cause oxygen deprivation, as can a tendency to form small clots.

All kinds of stress tend to make the liver sluggish. The liver normally removes toxins and excess hormones from the body. Estrogen can accumulate to high levels if the liver isn't fully active. One effect of estrogen is to promote oxidation of a type which doesn't provide energy, thus raising oxygen requirements. Another effect of estrogen is to inhibit a proteolytic enzyme in the blood, which normally dissolves clots. This is why birth control pills can cause blood clotting, strokes and other circulatory problems. Some of the long recognized signs of excessive estrogen are vascular "spiders," little red dots that some doctors like to burn off, brown spots on the skin, lumps in the breasts, a slight bluish color in some skin areas, puffiness, dizziness, etc.

Vitamin E promotes oxidation in many ways, and seems to specifically oppose many of the effects of excess estrogen. For example, it can help protect the liver against damage by toxins (all the nutrients are needed by the liver though). It opposes the tendency of estrogen to create "age pigment." It activates the blood protease, and so speeds clot removal and prevents clot formation inside blood vessels, but there is also evidence that it promotes normal clotting in wounds. The products of dissolving the proteins of clots are small peptide molecules called kinins, which act as local hormones to relax the walls of blood vessels, allowing easier flow of blood, better oxygenation, and lower blood pressure. Inside the cells, vitamin E inhibits destructive and wasteful oxidation (such as is involved in aging and cancer) and makes the normal oxidative process more efficient, providing more useful energy for a given amount of oxygen.

One theory of vitamin E action is that it protects progesterone. A recent discovery is that a prostaglandin (a hormone made from fatty acids) regulates blood pressure via the kidney — vitamin E protects fatty acids.

Recently it has been found that some natural vitamin E is contaminated with estrogen from the plant source, e.g., alfalfa.

Part of the reason for the common medical disbelief in the efficacy of vitamin E is that it doesn't work like a drug — a big dose doesn't immediately force the blood pressure down. Sometimes, in fact, the first effect is to strengthen a damaged heart, raising the blood pressure for a few days. But it does eventually remove many of the causes of high blood pressure, and I have never seen it fail to lower high blood pressure. Synthetic vitamin E is dl-alpha tocopherol, and may be associated with the reports of fatigue and headache from 800 units a day (however, this often repeated rumor is hard to track down — sort of like stories of blindness from vitamin A or LSD). Some "natural" vitamin E brands are contaminated with the petroleum distillate used for extraction, and taste like kerosene; the name d-alpha tocopherol indicates that it has been extracted from natural oils and has the "handedness" (chirality) of most biological substances (d and l mean right and left).

Other vitamins that can improve circulation by opening the small blood vessels are folic acid and niacin. Vitamin C can help to eliminate toxins that could contribute to high blood pressure. Trace minerals (such as those found in kelp and bran) and magnesium should also be considered in circulatory problems. Magnesium acts against calcium (and estrogen) in the clotting system, can prevent spasms of blood vessels, and can spare oxygen.

According to Barnes, nearly all hypertension can be helped with thyroid.

4. SOME DISEASES

NEARSIGHTEDNESS (MYOPIA)

Many years ago, I noticed that my nearsightedness increased when I was under stress. Many people become slightly nearsighted at night, or in the dark. Since the blood sugar concentration decreases at night, and under certain stress conditions, I guessed that myopia might be caused by chronic deficiency of sugar supply to the eye. This idea was reinforced when I read that tears normally contain more glucose than do the other body fluids, and then found that my tears usually had less sugar than the eyes of people with normal vision or with farsightedness. I found that many people (not just diabetic, whose altered refraction is usually blamed on swelling of the eyeball) had experienced very rapid and large changes in their degree of nearsightedness. In young women, I found that it was very common for them to become myopic within weeks of the time they began taking birth control pills, and that their vision sometimes corrected itself when they stopped taking the pill after a year or two. In women who were on the pill, and then began taking thyroid hormone, the thyroxin tended to correct their vision. Since estrogen tends to lower the blood sugar level, and thyroxin tends to raise it, these observations are consistent with the idea that myopia is caused by a deficiency of glucose in the eye. In the walls of the eyes of chickens, cells which look like smooth muscle cells are present. If smooth muscles in the wall of the eyeball are responsible for maintaining the roundness of the eye, against the near-focus apparatus around the lens, then chronic starvation of those cells would lead to elongation of the eyeball (in proportion to the amount of close work), producing myopia. Besides avoiding the pill, all of the anti-estrogen and anti-stress nutrients should help to prevent the progression of myopia, and being outside in good weather — to promote the tear flow — might even reverse it, as thyroid hormone does.

COLITIS, REGIONAL ENTERITIS (CROHN'S DISEASE), INFLAMMATION, AND FIBROUS DISEASES, AND "COLLAGEN DISEASE"

Stress consumes steroids and produces the many degenerative diseases described by Hans Selye. The gastro-intestinal system becomes inflamed or ulcerated, and fibrous tissue may proliferate. Adrenal glands enlarge, and lymphoid tissue shrinks during the first stage of stress (and may enlarge later). Stress can be produced by dark cloudy northern winters, by inadequate nutrition, by the use of estrogen and many other drugs, and by the use of foods which inhibit the thyroid gland (bakery bread, lacking available manganese and containing iodate and bromate; cabbage family, and many cereals and nuts containing nitriles, cyanide or thiocyanate; meats "refined" from animals whose thyroid tissue is sold to drug companies).

Stress diseases typically have a dominant allergic aspect, and respond to steroids. Cortisone is used medically, but has side effects which could be avoided by using progesterone (though "medical" progesterone usually contains allergenic solvents and "preservatives" such as phenol). Niacin, vitamin A, vitamin C, etc., help to produce progesterone, and so often help in stress diseases, though the manufactured substances are themselves somewhat allergenic. (Vitamin A is not usually "manufactured.")

Light deprivation can be remedied artificially, but the necessary brightness is usually underestimated. Because an adequate diet is hard to get in our culture, which makes it *illegal* to sell the thyroid gland as food, it is often necessary to buy this powdered meat in tablet form from your physician and druggist. Meat eaters would normally get 1/4 to 1/2 grain of thyroid in their food every day if the whole animal were used. Eggs, sardines, oysters, chicken stew (non-estrogenized chickens), etc., are examples of 'unrefined" protein foods which shouldn't interfere with thyroid function. Vegetarians often notice temporary exhilaration when they stop eating meat, probably because their thyroid has been suppressed. But a more serious hypothyroid state often follows, from a low protein inadequate vegetarian diet. Low protein diets definitely interfere with the liver's ability to detoxify estrogen and other stressors.

A diet high in animal protein with other nutrients, including an appropriate amount of desiccated thyroid if "refined" proteins are used, can cause an immediate improvement in many diseases which are specifically produced by stress.

HEART DISEASE

There are several reasons to suspect that a magnesium deficiency is often involved in heart disease; in a clinical study, for example, injected magnesium sulphate helped in angina pectoris and coronary thrombosis, and tended to lower blood lipids. Numerous studies have found that a high magnesium intake is associated with low blood cholesterol levels. Magnesium also opposes clot formation and vascular spasm, which can be promoted by an excess of calcium. Estrogen was once used to "prevent" heart attacks, but it is now known to *induce* heart attacks in both men and women. Vascular spasm is now recognized as a cause of heart attacks.

The Shutes have done extensive research on the use of vitamin E in heart disease, and found that "pharmacological" doses of 400 mg/day or more are beneficial. They have also recommended it for preventing thrombosis elsewhere in the vascular system. In problems such as varicose veins and clots in the legs, they say:

> It mobilizes collateral or detour circulation about the obstructed veins in the deep parts of the leg. It is the best and safest agent one can use. It not only melts away the existing clot and helps the inflammatory process to subside, but it hinders

> extension of that process and almost never permits a part of the clot to break loose and strike some other part of the body, such as the lungs or brain (an accident called embolism). We feel that vitamin E is very effective in preventing thrombosis within the vascular system, and acts more simply, more cheaply and much more safely than the rival anticoagulants.

Other points relating to heart disease are discussed in the section on high blood pressure. Low thyroid is known to be a cause of both heart attacks and of elevated blood cholesterol. (B. Barnes; Adv. in Lipid Res.)

ARTERIOSCLEROSIS

The American Dietetic Association warns about overdosing with kelp, because of the iodide; but the Japanese eat various iodide-rich seaweeds without the thyroid problems the A.D.A. says might occur on the kelp-lecithin-vinegar B6 diet. In the U.S. people who eat bakery bread receive about 10 times more than the RDA of iodine. Iodides are known to benefit arteriosclerosis, with visible improvement occurring in blood vessels in the retina (see *Physicians Desk Reference,* iodides). In old age, the walls of blood vessels tend to become hardened with calcium. In at least some tissues, it is known that calcification begins in degenerating mitochondria, and mitochondria tend to deteriorate in aging tissue. Nutrients such as iodine, vitamin E, magnesium and vitamin B2 are especially important for maintaining the function of the mitochondria, which produce most of our energy. An excess of iodine from bread or kelp is much more likely to interfere with the thyroid when the diet contains a large amount of unsaturated fat, such as safflower or soy oil, because these combine with iodine to form substances which inhibit the thyroid. These oils in themselves suppress the thyroid, and this might be a factor in the premature aging and increased cancer rate which have been observed in people who use larger amounts of those oils.

Atherosclerotic damage (fatty deposits) of blood vessels is made worse by sugar supposedly, since insulin is involved in cholesterol damage. There is evidence that lecithin and other phospholipids protect the body against fatty degeneration. Eggs, for several reasons might actively protect against the formation of cholesterol deposits. One of the men who discovered insulin, Best, later showed that choline (a component of lecithin) can prevent fatty degeneration of the liver. Very large doses of biotin cause experimental animals to develop fatty livers (developing into liver cancer), but this effect can be offset by feeding the animal another B vitamin, inositol. Some of these effects have been known for about half a century, but too many "health professionals" are still pretending that no valid data exist. Maybe we should start asking whether these "health professionals" have a valid existence.

POLIO: A CHRONOLOGY (OR, ISN'T SCIENCE WONDERFUL?)

Muller in Switzerland in 1830 built the steel roller wheat mill.

Jacob von Heine first diagnosed polio, 1840.

First polio epidemic, Sweden, 1887.

Epidemic in some region of U.S. almost every year after 1900.

In 1952, epidemics in Denmark, Germany, Belgium, 33,344 cases in U.S.

An epidemic of rumors that Mexicans didn't get polio because of the absence of white bread and sugar in their country. (Sugar refining developed in Europe roughly parallel with flour refining.) The white flour producers financed research by a Harvard group to find the cause of Mexicans' apparent resistance to polio. The Harvard scientists concluded that Mexicans are so dirty that they are constantly eating the polio virus and so never catch the disease.

According to Harrison's *Principles of Internal Medicine,* polio can be spread by injection, including vaccination. Salk vaccine in many cases apparently brought on polio after the first or second injection in the series of three. Studies in which people were advised to avoid sugar and starch during the (summer) "polio season" never got government or institutional support. However, some studies were done: see the section on infections.

MULTIPLE SCLEROSIS

Roger MacDougall's diet for preventing the progression of multiple sclerosis involves avoidance of gluten and the use of a vitamin-mineral supplement. A letter in *The Lancet* (Oct. 5, 1974) describes one form of the diet: "subject avoids eating wheat, oats, rye and barley...takes less saturated fat, replacing it in part by unsaturated fat, reduces his sugar intake, replacing the remaining white sugar by Barbados sugar, and supplements his intake of food with" the following:

Vitamin B1	24 mg. (per day)
Vitamin B2	12 mg.
Vitamin B6	60 mg.
Nicotinamide	1 gram
Calcium Pantothenate	120 mg.
Vitamin C	600 mg.
Vitamin E	180 mg.
Calcium gluconate	900 mg.
Magnesium hydroxide	900 mg.
Vitamin B12	150 micrograms

That writer suggests that the calcium might not be desirable in the formula. I think the magnesium is extremely important, and it might be better to use it in a more soluble form, such as magnesium carbonate or magnesium chloride, or even epsom salts (magnesium sulphate) which in large doses can't be absorbed, but in small doses will be partly converted to the chloride by stomach acid. Some people, suspected of having early MS, have been able to stop the symptoms just by avoiding carbohydrates. Biotin is involved in the synthesis of fats in the nervous system, and so should probably be given special attention in the MS diet. Liver is a good source of it. If it is taken as a supplement, inositol (and probably choline) should be taken with it, because large doses of biotin by itself were toxic in animal experiments.

Stress, the immune system, and lipid metabolism have complex interactions. For example, a fat, triolein, is known to stimulate phagocytosis, as does magnesium; sugar in the diet has an opposite effect. Stress increases breakdown of fats, and can decrease the proportion of triglycerides (triolein is a triglyceride, meaning it is composed of glycerin and three fatty acid molecules) in the blood. Avoiding stress (coffee, tea, and other stimulants produce a stress-like reaction in many people) should be part of a multiple sclerosis program.

Steroids have been used apparently to inhibit an inflammatory process, though it was about 1978 before an active brain inflammation was observed in a person who died with MS. Good nutrition would support the synthesis of natural steroids. Hypothyroidism can mimic the neurological problems of MS, but neurologists are generally willing to diagnose a condition as MS without giving thyroid tests. Vitamin A is needed for steroid production and should be added to MacDougall's program. I think beans and nuts should be avoided as well as the grains.

Polyunsaturated oils inhibit the immune system and so probably suppress symptoms. The steroids (e.g., progesterone) and thyroid hormones normalize the immune system when they are present in normal amounts.

INFECTIONS

In the winter of 1974, a young professor visited me to talk about Blake College, and we started talking about nutrition and health. After I told him some stories about antibiotics and vitamin A, he mentioned that he had a chronic, active and uncomfortable infection of the urethra (non-specific urethritis, a bacterial infection of the urinary canal, usually involving E. coli, the common intestinal bacteria, and less often Proteus, Staphylococcus aureus, Enterobacter, Pseudomonas, etc.) for nearly two years. Twice he had been given a month's course of high potency antibiotics, which suppressed the symptoms while he continued to take them, but the condition returned immediately when he stopped taking the antibiotics. He was interested in trying to nutritionally raise his immunity, so I gave him liver for lunch, and suggested that he eat some daily, and gave him a week's supply of vitamins A, E, folic acid, B6, potassium and magnesium. He was scheduled to come back to town in a week, so I asked him to let me know how he felt then. About a day later, he came back in a very surprised state, and said the infection had already completely cleared up. This spring (1975) he came back and is still free of the infection. This sort of infection is more common in women, and usually takes longer to clear up.

Folic acid, known for its ability to cure some anemias (red blood cell deficiency) also improves the function of white blood cells, improving antibody production. It is also possibly involved in a non-antibody process which allows white blood cells to destroy virus, fungi, and other parasites. Vitamin A, besides strengthening membranes, is necessary for protein synthesis, and so helps form the immune tissue. Zinc has similar general functions in protein antibody production, but also possibly has a direct "viricidal" capacity, as observed *in vitro,* which would account for its release (and loss) during viral infections. Vitamin A (and possibly folic acid) mediate the body's response to light, and so modify its neural control of immunity, thyroid and adrenal and sex hormone function, etc.

Unsaturated fatty acids inhibit some immune functions and also inhibit the thyroid gland and directly inhibit cellular respiration. As Broda Barnes has pointed out, hypothyroidism predisposes people to infections; chronic respiratory, ear, and bladder infections are common results.

Vitamin C increases the structural strength of the mucous membranes' connective tissue, in proportion to its intake, up to the mega-doses recommended by Pauling (according to electron microscope evidence, *J. Clin. Nutr.*, summer, 1974). It is also more concentrated in white blood cells than in any other tissue (about a 60 to one ratio between white blood cells and surrounding fluids), and their immune function depends on its presence in adequate amounts. Up to 200 mg. daily intake, vitamin C concentration in blood and tissues increases rapidly, and the kidneys work to reabsorb it; at about that intake, the kidney's ability to conserve it becomes "saturated", so that higher doses are retained at lower efficiency. The increased body retention of vitamin C when 5 grams per day is taken is about 4 times that of 100 mg. per day.

Zinc and vitamin A may also act through the blood sugar. It is well known that an emotional upset, spending too much time in the sun, working too long without eating, etc., can bring on an attack of herpes ("cold sores", for example): low blood sugar probably precipitates the eruption. Polio outbreaks always occurred in the summer when people tend to eat more carbohydrate (because of the lower specific dynamic action, relative to protein — it heats the body less for a given amount of energy). B.F. Sandler wrote a book on nutrition for avoiding polio (H.G. Muller-Verlag, Krailling bei Munchen, 1959) in which he claimed that infection with the polio virus is only possible if the blood sugar goes below 80 mg. per cent. If this is true of the herpes virus, it would suggest a reason for the association of cancer with both herpes and estrogen, since estrogen lowers blood sugar, and both the virus and estrogen can cause tissue irritation and cell division. Vitamin A is being used experimentally to prevent cancer and to reverse precancerous conditions, especially in the cervix and the mouth. Many women have premenstrual herpes outbreaks which can be controlled with progesterone or thyroid.

P. Delbet used physiological magnesium chloride (12.1 grams per liter) to stimulate phagocytosis in white blood cells. The activity was more than doubled by injection of 150 cc. of this solution into a dog, or by application to cells in vitro. (See *Magnesium: the Nutrient that Could Change Your Life,* J.I. Rodale, Pyramid, New York, 1968.) Dr. U.D. Register, of the School of Health at Loma Linda University, has done related work that shows a decline of white blood cell activity with increased sugar in the diet.

CHRONIC FATIGUE

Various researchers have found that the cells of fat, or depressed, or tired people are in a low energy state, and, increasingly, it is being recognized that this low energy state resembles hypothyroidism. Many things can cause hypothyroidism--too much estrogen or cortisol, too little progesterone, a diet containing too little good quality protein, too few calories, or diets containing significant quantities of beans, lentils, or undercooked broccoli or cauliflower—but in our culture unsaturated oils are probably the most important cause.

As early as 1951, it was known (Kunkel and Williams, J. Biol. Chem.) that the polyunsaturated fatty acids strongly inhibit the crucial respiratory enzyme, cytochrome oxidase, and that inhibition of this enzyme has a very important effect on the whole animal, suppressing its metabolic rate, reducing the number of calories it can burn.

It is now known that polyunsaturated fats interfere with thyroid hormone in just about every conceivable way.

One of the most common symptoms of hypothyroidism is lethargy, fatigue that persists even while getting extra rest and sleep. Everything is inefficient in hypothyroidism, even sleep. Occasionally, a low thyroid person can compensate for the basic metabolic defect by producing very large amounts of adrenalin. These people seem to have excess energy, and sometimes need less sleep than average, but on the level of tissue function, they are similar to the chronically fatigued people, being slow to produce energy. Compensating for low thyroid with high adrenalin creates specific metabolic problems, including circulatory and heart disease. Slow relaxation of muscles, caused by respiratory inhibition, can produce chronic soreness and stiffness, which is a common feature of the "chronic fatigue syndrome."

Cold fingers and toes are one of the most common signs of hypothyroidism, and result from a low rate of metabolic heat production, combined with the effects of adrenalin, restricting blood flow to the extremities to preserve the body's limited heat. Experimenters have found that sodium tends to increase body temperature, and eating additional salt sometimes helps to break out of the low energy hypothyroid state; one effect of extra salt is that it makes it easier for the body to retain its magnesium, which is very closely associated with cellular energy.

All animals respond to the stressful effects of reduced sunshine in winter with adjustments in their thyroid functions. Typically, mammals need several times as much thyroid during the winter as they do in the summer. If a person is taking a balanced thyroid supplement, increasing the dose is often all it takes to avoid the lethargy, weight gain, and "seasonal affective disorder" that often occurs in the winter. A variety of stress-related diseases tend to get worse during the winter, and sometimes they make their first appearance in the winter. The rate of aging is greatest in the winter, and the risk of death is highest. All of the protective hormones tend to fall during the winter.

On pages 153 and 161, I have added two new charts that schematically show the relation of thyroid hormones and other factors to the protective and youth associated steroid hormones.

FOOD ALLERGIES

Cooking, by altering the proteins, can lower the allergic reaction to many foods. Soaking seeds before cooking them can have the same effect. Storing foods such as seeds in a sealed bottle in the refrigerator will slow the deterioration of oils, and rancid oils can be very toxic and irritating. Many people lose their allergies (even hay fever and poison-oak sensitivity) when they take supplements of the vitamins A, C, and pantothenic acid.

Heat will destroy some seed toxins, but it also creates new poisons and damages the protein quality. For example, heat cause lysine to react with sugars, forming a carcinogen.

Plants evolved special toxins to protect their seeds from animals, so "seed poisoning" is probably a more accurate description than "allergy to grains, nuts, legumes, seeds." Low thyroid function leads to poor digestion and to hypoglycemia, both of which make an allergic reaction more likely.

A NOTE ON GLAUCOMA

Because of their stress-like effects, coffee and tobacco should be avoided in glaucoma. The nutrients that are especially involved in the adrenal stress reaction should be used: ascorbic acid, pantothenic acid, riboflavin, vitamin A, magnesium, and vitamin E.

Progesterone (natural form) is a diuretic and also is a precursor for the anti-stress hormones, and sometimes helps glaucoma. The nutrients mentioned above promote its synthesis. Estrogen blocks its actions, so it would seem desirable to avoid estrogen, and to use the nutrients which oppose estrogen.

The eye itself has especially high requirements for vitamins A, B2, and niacin, and coenzyme Q.

Salt and water metabolism involve vitamins B6, pantothenic acid, A, C, E, and niacin (see R.J. Kutsky, *Handbook of Vitamins and Hormones,* p. 263), and various minerals (other than sodium) including magnesium, potassium and zinc.

Because of the role of carbon dioxide in circulation, vitamins B1, B6, and biotin, and zinc, should also be considered. Choline is now known to stimulate acetylcholine synthesis, and so might help to promote a normal parasympathetic innervation.

INSOMNIA

A few weeks ago, a woman, in her 40s and taking estrogen pills by prescription, was complaining of extreme insomnia and other symptoms. I suggested that she might be getting too much estrogen, so she stopped, and immediately was able to sleep normally. Sometimes a few hundred milligrams of magnesium carbonate per day (or a spoonful of epsom salts, if this dose is divided into several parts to avoid the laxative effect) will immediately make it possible to sleep normally. Zinc, as in oysters, and potassium and the B complex vitamins, as in brewer's yeast, are sometimes necessary. Many people get gas from the complex carbohydrates in yeast. This can be prevented by steeping a tablespoonful in a cup of boiling water, and drinking only the yellow liquid and throwing away the sediment. Protein is lost, but the other nutrients are highly soluble. Milk contains natural sleep-inducers, including the amino acid tryptophan and milk sugar. Two or three tablespoonfuls of honey in a glass of milk will provide some magnesium, as well as sugar to increase the liver's stored glycogen. When blood sugar is low, adrenalin is secreted to raise the sugar level, but it also tends to keep the person awake, by causing nightmares, sweating, rapid heartbeat, etc. Since blood sugar is normally higher in the daytime, because of light's effect on various glands, some people with defective livers find it easier to sleep in the daytime. Hypothyroidism is the most common basic cause of low blood sugar, and very commonly causes insomnia. I have noticed that "bedtime worries" are associated with hypothyroidism, and disappear when it is corrected.

Although tryptophan supplements are available for insomnia, I think its chronic use would be as dangerous as the tranquilizer, reserpine, which acts on the same biochemical system, and which increases the risk of breast cancer.

LOW BLOOD PRESSURE

Some doctors say that lower than average blood pressure is a good thing. Many women have a systolic pressure of around 100, and I think rightly suspect that it relates to their feelings of weakness or fatigue or even dizziness. Sometimes orthostatic hypotension, the failure of blood pressure to rise when the person stands up, is described as "dizziness." A relative deficiency of the catecholamines can produce these symptoms.

For several years I had suspected a connection between estrogen and low blood pressure, just from noticing that women with seemingly high estrogen tended to have lower than average blood pressure. The fact that estrogen, acting as an antagonist to vitamin E, could promote high blood pressure had distracted my attention from the opposite effect, being produced by an antagonism to thyroxin. It was enough of a heresy, for the moment, to point out the many ways in which estrogen antagonizes thyroxin; in addition to things I have mentioned elsewhere, I think the opposition is also visible in the action of estrogen on blood lipids. Since aging and x-rays have some biochemical effects similar to those of estrogen, they might also antagonize thyroxin; this suggests that large doses of thyroxin might be used in senility, radiation sickness, and cancer.

Since thyroxine potentiates adrenalin, which maintains blood pressure, excess estrogen, antagonizing thyroid, could tend to lower blood pressure through this system. The thermogenic effect of progesterone might act by way of thyroxin; if so, it might be the best way of counteracting estrogen and promoting thyroxin activity. The opposite reaction to high estrogen-low thyroid is also known to occur: an elevation of brain catecholamines and also an elevation of blood pressure. Thus, a thyroid supplement can often correct hypertension, as well as hypotension.

SKIN FEEDING

Oily things enter the body very easily through the skin. Toxic solvents should never touch the skin, just as they never should be breathed. Oily vitamins and hormones can be applied to the skin. There is a form of vitamin C (ascorbic palmitate) which enters the skin quickly, and according to the Soviet researchers who developed it, can be used to carry other nutrients in through the skin. Significant quantities of fat (such as olive oil) can be given by massage when the person is too sick to eat. For years people have noticed that zinc oxide ointment speeds healing, just as zinc in the diet improves healing. Zinc chloride dissolved in vegetable oil was found to raise blood zinc very effectively when painted onto the skin. Zinc has been used successfully to treat stretch marks. Probably other minerals will enter the skin as easily — magnesium sulphate (epsom salts) is a traditional treatment for inflammations. Since carbon dioxide dissolves best in "oil loving" material such as the skin, it enters the body even against a concentration gradient. Adding baking soda to an epsom salts soak should make it more effective. Mineral oil, vaseline, and rancid vegetable oil should not be put on the skin. Lotions and other cosmetics generally contain mineral oil.

IDENTIFYING DEFICIENCIES

Frequent nosebleeds, bloodshot eyes. and visible blood vessels on the cheeks and nose can be symptoms of a deficiency of vitamin B2. Vitamin C, rutin, and iodide are other nutrients that can sometimes correct blood vessel problems.

A peculiar kind of irritability, sometimes with a sense of having your head in a kind of "cloud", is often a result of a vitamin B1 deficiency. If that is the cause, it will clear up within a few minutes after taking the vitamin. Magnesium deficiency is another common cause of irritability.

White stripes across the fingernails, especially on the right hand, seem to represent a zinc deficiency. Menstruation can cause loss of zinc, so that some women have five or six spots evenly spaced up the length of the nail, each resulting from one period. The length of the nail represents about six months' growth. A virus infection can have the same effect. The eyebrows sometimes become bristly in a zinc deficiency. A zinc deficiency is often associated with a deficiency of vitamin B6 and an excess of copper; since estrogen is associated with zinc loss, other nutrients including vitamin E and folic acid should be considered when the nails have white marks.

Sore spots at the sides of the mouth often result from a vitamin B2 deficiency; other B vitamin deficiencies can cause a sore tongue, and a niacin or protein deficiency can show up first in the gums as tenderness or bleeding. (A thyroid deficiency contributes to receding and bleeding gums, pyorrhea, etc. A recent book on Ubiquinone, coenzyme Q, shows that gums heal rapidly when the person consumes a ubiquinone supplement. This nutrient is found in heart, liver, greens, etc., and is closely related to both vitamin E and thyroid hormones.)

Teeth that are sensitive to heat or cold suggest a deficiency of calcium, magnesium, or vitamin D. Blood sugar and calcium seem to be related, and a dental researcher has shown that teeth are sensitive to alterations in the blood sugar concentration. Cramps, especially in the feet and legs can result from a deficiency of these same nutrients.

Weak fingernails are common in protein deficiency and hypothyroidism. Falling or very fine hair also suggest hypothyroidism, which can result from stress or eating antithyroid foods. Many other symptoms are discussed in sections on progesterone, thyroid and estrogen.

WARBURG'S CANCER THEORY, CACHEXIA AND THYROID THERAPY

Warburg[1] demonstrated that all cancers have defective respiration, by which he meant that glucose is consumed too rapidly. The excessive consumption of glucose in the presence of oxygen is called aerobic glycolysis, and is typical of cancer. Oxygen may be consumed, but it does not result in the production of sufficient ATP to inhibit glycolysis (by the Pasteur Effect). This generally means that excess lactate will be produced and will leave the cell, will be detected by other tissues, and will be processed by the liver into glucose. Lactate is a sufficient stimulus to trigger the stress reaction, and in many people causes an anxiety syndrome. Since resynthesis of glucose from lactate by the liver requires much more energy than is derived from conversion of glucose to lactate, the tumor's formation of lactate constitutes a large energy burden to the organism. Total energy consumption would increase, because of intense but inefficient metabolism in the tumor and in the liver, and also possibly because of stress-induced brain excitation and the catabolism of muscle and other tissue proteins. Cortisone elevates blood glucose and would inhibit the thyroid. Since there is evidence of thyroid deficiency in various cancers, and since thyroid supplementation reduces the incidence of spontaneous tumors, thyroid therapy would be desirable in cancer, especially if there is cachexia. Gerson[2] and Tallberg[3] have reported good results from using thyroid as part of supportive therapy.

The stereotype of the hypothyroid person as overweight will lead the typical physician to believe that metabolic stimulation by thyroid would be exactly the opposite of what the cachectic patient needs. The relevant effects of thyroid (especially with progesterone, to promote tissue response to thyroid, and to block cortisone production) however, are stimulation of protein synthesis and the prevention of lactate formation - or the stimulation of its oxidation, either by the tumor itself or by other tissues, to prevent its entry into the Cori cycle, for gluconeogenesis. (Cachexia strumipriva should be kept in mind).

Warburg believed that a riboflavin deficiency was an important contributor to the development of defective respiration, but he also pointed out that the simple lack of oxygen would promote the development of cancer. I have emphasized the role of estrogen in creating an oxygen deficiency. Since it inhibits the secretion of thyroxin at the glandular level, and antagonizes thyroxin at the cellular level, estrogen is a good candidate for the main cause of the respiratory defect. It also antagonizes other respiratory factors, such as magnesium and vitamin E, and radioactive estrogen has been shown to accumulate selectively in (liver) cancer cells. (And excess estrogen actually impedes oxygenation of the blood.)

Once we accept Warburg's thesis, that damaged respiration is the prime cause of cancer, the therapeutic use of thyroid in cancer seems obvious. Schizophrenics seem to have either a resistance to thyroid hormones or an inability to convert T4 to T3. Aging and estrogen dominance are other states in which cells seem to be relatively insensitive to thyroid hormones. If the liver is a main site of T4's conversion to T3, cancer patients may require very large doses of thyroid, or else direct use of T3 (possibly in large doses), since the liver is so likely to be inefficient.

[1]Otto Heinrich Warburg, **The Metabolism of Tumors,** R.R. Smith, Inc., New York, 1931.

[2]Max Gerson, **A Cancer Therapy,** Whitier Books, New York, 1958.

[3] Tallberg, **Protides of the Body Fluids,** 1978.

CANCER, STRESS, AND NUTRITION: A SUMMARY

Cancer lives on sugar. It disturbs metabolism, tending to lower blood sugar (even to the point of causing hallucinations) and promotes the conversion of good tissue into sugar: the liver and the immune tissue are the first to show this effect. Stress first elevates adrenaline, which causes fear and anxiety; adrenaline then stimulates the body to produce cortisone. If nutrients, especially vitamins C and A, are available the adrenal glands will produce cortisone to maintain the blood sugar as long as some good body tissue remains to convert to sugar, unless adaptation occurs.

If the body can adapt to get most of its energy from fat oxidation, then blockage of sugar metabolism can lead to starvation of the cancer. A magnesium deficiency damages energy production and leads to high sugar consumption, with the associated tendency to destroy protein. During healthy adaptation to fasting, the body consumes fat preferentially — the brain is usually the biggest consumer of glucose, and it can adapt in about two weeks to oxidize mainly fat, as ketones. In this state, the kidneys (as well as any cancer) will consume protein and produce ammonia and fuel; the kidneys synthesize glucose (estimated at roughly 40 grams per day) from the protein, but the reason for this reaction seems to be the need for ammonium ions to balance the keto acids which are being eliminated in the urine. If the need for positive ions regulates this conversion of protein to glucose, then the wasting of the body and the production of glucose could be reduced even more by providing positive ions — as carbonates, or carbonate precursors to be chosen by their tendency to stimulate respiration rather than gluconeogenesis (possibly citrate or acetate, though acetate might inhibit lipolysis; these anions would be needed in such small amounts that their effects might be negligible). The cations would be chosen for their ability to regulate many aspects of metabolism, including glycolysis, respiration, hormone secretion, and immunity. They would include, in order of probable quantities, magnesium, zinc, manganese, and molybdenum. Certain fruits probably approximate the ionic balance needed.

Very high elevations produce hormonal and metabolic adaptations which are appropriate for recovery from cancer. (See S. Tromp's *Medical Biometeorology,* and F.Z. Meyerson's work in the Soviet Union.) Even moderate increases in elevation lower the cancer rate (see references in my article on the "excitable ether").

Vitamin A is needed for proper differentiation of various types of cell, and has been used successfully in blocking cancer formation and in causing precancerous tissue to return to normal. Progesterone "spares" vitamin A, and has been used in cancer therapy. Iodine has a long history of use in cancer therapy; the tissue lump produced by tuberculosis bacilli has some similarity to tumor formation in cancer (this was an idea behind the use of a harmless form of the tuberculosis organism, BCG, in cancer therapy to stimulate the immune rejection system). Iodine was found to restore activity to proteolytic enzymes which are inhibited by TB, and allow dissolution of the nodule. Progesterone and vitamin A interact with the thyroid hormone; when body temperature is below normal

there is typically a progesterone deficiency (or estrogen excess, which may be functionally equivalent to a thyroid deficiency). Normal inhibitors of cell division (chalones) are not retained in cells at a normal level when ATP and vitamin E are deficient. Rapid growth is obviously one factor which could make it difficult to obtain adequate levels of some nutrients, such as the oily vitamins A, K, E, and D, just as wasteful use of oxygen can rob adjacent tissues and lead to spreading of the inflammation. ATP normally circulates in the blood in amounts reflecting cellular efficiency. Just as rigor mortis can be softened by injection of ATP, the hardness of a tumor probably reflects ATP deficiency (softening of cervical tumors was observed during progesterone treatment). Intravenous ATP (it could be purified by patient's own serum proteolytic enzyme before use to avoid immune reaction) should be considered as part of a physiological therapy.
Magnesium salt of ATP is the appropriate form.

Intravenous ethanol prevents protein wastage without providing glucose to feed cancer; it controls pain as well as morphine with less toxicity. It can also be used as a skin rub, again bypassing the liver. Magnesium carbonate can be given by any route, though it would have to be buffered intravenously. (5% ethanol has been used intravenously, safely.)

Pyrroles and porphyrins in blood and urine, if elevated, suggest that therapies should continue, even if symptoms have disappeared.

Nutrition through the skin can be significant in cancer: oils, vitamins, and minerals go into the skin easily, especially when they are applied in an oily medium.

THE CERVICAL CANCER SCARE

Many women with abnormal Pap smears, even with a biopsy showing the so-called "carcinoma *in situ,*" have returned to normal in just two months with a diet including the following: 90 grams of protein, 500 mg. of magnesium as the chloride, 100,000 units of vitamin A, 400 units of vitamin E, 5 mg. of folic acid, 100 mg. of pantothenic acid, 100 mg. of B6, 100 mg. of niacinamide, and 500 mg. of vitamin C, with thyroid and progesterone as needed. Liver should be eaten twice a week. Some of the women apply vitamin A directly to the cervix.

ASTHMA, MIGRAINE, PSORIASIS

During LSD research, it was noticed that people with chronic headaches, asthma, or psoriasis sometimes recovered completely during treatment with frequent doses of LSD. Another alkaloid derived from ergot, bromocriptine, is now being used to suppress lactation (such as is caused by prolactin-secreting pituitary tumor which develops after using oral contraceptives) and is used experimentally to treat Parkinson's disease. Both LSD and bromocriptine shift the ratio of two brain chemicals, DOPA and serotonin, towards DOPA dominance. Among the effects of this is an inhibition of prolactin secretion. Prolactin excess is involved in breast cancer and in other cell proliferation, probably including the rapid cell division in psoriasis. Prolactin apparently inhibits progesterone production, and so could establish a self-stimulating vicious circle. All of the effects of prolactin excess (including amenorrhea) which respond to an increase of the DOPA/ serotonin ratio can be obtained to some extent by other, more easily available, materials. Vitamin B6, thyroid, and progesterone all have this action. Nickel has been found to have this effect in animals, but isn't available as a nutritional supplement. Thyroid and progesterone have relieved asthma, migraine and psoriasis (or eczema) very effectively. Since tryptophan, an amino acid which is being promoted as a sedative, causes an increase of serotonin in the brain, it should not be used as a supplement by people with any of these "low DOPA" symptoms. Milk is a rich natural source of tryptophan. Since tryptophan promotes formation of serotonin which stimulates release of prolactin, and prolactin activates the formation of sebum (oil) by the skin, large amounts of milk could promote a tendency toward acne, when there is a deficiency of B6, thyroid, progesterone, etc.

Although the prolactin-secreting pituitary tumor was very rare a few years ago, it is now the most common form of pituitary tumor. In the 1930's Korenchevsky demonstrated that estrogen produced that kind of tumor, among many others, and that the tumor would regress under the influence of progesterone. Since the liver requires adequate protein to eliminate estrogen, a low protein diet or other deficiencies would undoubtedly contribute to the development of this tumor in a user of birth control pills. Estrogen stimulates cell division in the prolactin-secreting part of the pituitary, and elevates the level of serotonin, and so can be the basic chemical cause of these various symptoms. Diet, stress, and amount of light, of course, can modify the level of estrogen and its actions. The avoidance of anti-thyroid foods such as soy beans, cabbage, and peanuts would be especially important.

5. PREGNANCY AND CHILDREN

AGE AND PREGNANCY

Women are often encouraged to have their children while they are young, by the fear of having a Mongoloid baby (Down's syndrome), which happens more often in older mothers. But someone did a study that showed that Mongoloids are borne more often by women who have been married longer. Women who marry at 30 or 35, for example, were found to have fewer Mongoloid babies than women of the same age who had married younger. The investigator suggested that long-married couples so seldom made love that the chances were greater for the egg (or egg and sperm both) to deteriorate before being fertilized.

Other studies show teenage mothers have babies with smaller brains than average, and with a greater chance of being slightly retarded. (Smoking during pregnancy has the same effect; carbon monoxide in city air would probably contribute to the damage.) If women are encouraged to have babies younger, will the population have smaller brains?

Diabetic women are known to typically have large babies with big heads, who learn quickly. With each pregnancy, a woman tends to have less "glucose tolerance," or to seem more diabetic. HCG, the hormone which helps sustain pregnancy, raises the blood sugar to meet the fetus's need for abundant sugar. So diabetes and pregnancy have much in common. And as a woman gets older she tends towards diabetes, and so tends to nourish the fetus better, especially its brain. Besides this natural tendency, a more mature woman is less likely to live on snack foods.

The results of these studies indicate that later marriage would help to reduce the number of mentally retarded children. And better nutrition before and during pregnancy and nursing makes a great difference in the baby's mental and physical development. Young women who are pregnant should be especially careful to avoid low blood sugar. Older women will probably require a little more vitamin E, and should be especially sure that they aren't getting a toxic amount of copper from their water supply or utensils. Regardless of age, pregnant women should make a special effort to get perfect nutrition every day, and to avoid poisons, including drugs, fumes and smoke. Even drugs which don't enter the fetus directly can affect its health by disturbing the mother's metabolism. Many drugs (and food additives) can increase a person's nutritional needs, for example by increasing the rate at which vitamin C is lost in the urine.

Recently there has been a great increase in sterility from endometriosis. Delayed reproduction is a suspected factor. A progesterone deficiency has been implicated. Thyroid, protein and vitamin A help to maintain progesterone production. Alcohol and other drugs used by the father can also cause birth defects.

PRECOCIOUS BABIES

Too much estrogen, insulin, unsaturated fats, or other things which tend to lower blood sugar (toxins including copper, stress, etc.) can lead to mentally retarded babies, premature and underweight babies, and small brained babies. Factors which help to maintain blood sugar, including good diet and hormones such as thyroxin and progesterone, help to produce big, healthy, large brained and precocious babies.

During the last few months of pregnancy, there is often a craving for sweet things, which should be satisfied with fruit. The potassium in fruit has an effect like that of insulin, so that sugar from the fruit can become available to cells without over-stimulating insulin secretion. Since insulin persists after disposing of excess sugar, it tends to keep blood sugar low and to intensify craving for carbohydrates.

Pantothenic acid helps to destroy insulin; this is one way it helps to maintain adequate blood sugar levels.

During pregnancy the mother's body adapts to live increasingly on fat, so that most of the sugar which is available can be used by the baby. The brain uses most of the body's glucose, so mental fatigue can easily affect the blood sugar level. The developing baby is extremely dependent on glucose for its energy supply, and its brain can be damaged by sugar starvation.

Women who are mildly diabetic are known to have big, precocious babies with large heads. Pregnancy itself resembles diabetes, in the adaptation to oxidizing fat rather than sugar, so that a slight tendency toward diabetes can be thought of as a support for pregnancy. Older women are more likely to have some degree of "diabetes," or elevated blood sugar. With each pregnancy, there is a tendency for the blood sugar to be higher, and for the baby to be bigger and more precocious. Older women, in fact, tend to have superior babies. However, after several pregnancies, especially if they are spaced so closely that the body doesn't have time to recover from the depletion of nutrients, the average birth weight suddenly falls, and problems of cell division such as twinning or Down's syndrome become much more common. The fact that the fourth or fifth baby is always borne by an "older" woman has led to the mistaken belief that age alone is responsible for "mongolism." The essential role of nutritional depletion is shown by comparing birth weights and birth defects in women of different social classes and incomes: at a given age, birth weights are lower and birth defects are more common, and the symptoms of depletion (loss of teeth, decreased birth weight, infertility) occur sooner in poor classes.

Vitamin E, vitamin A, and magnesium are other nutrients that help to maintain blood sugar. Vitamin B12 is needed to use vitamin A. Folic acid, vitamin B6, and zinc are depleted by elevated estrogen and are especially important for healthy pregnancy. Too much copper can lower blood sugar; too much iron can destroy vitamin E, and vitamin E deficiency can lead to jaundice, which can affect the baby's brain.

NUTRITION-RELATED IDEAS FOR MOTHERS

If you are sick, reconsider everything you are doing as a contributing factor. There is an ideology about sickness being "eliminative". This tends to produce some confusion, about sickness being healthy.

Give yourself time to get entirely well before getting pregnant. C. Brown-Sequard bred injured guinea pigs and found that the offspring had a high rate of epilepsy and birth defects. Sickness or trauma — including surgery — can bring on a chronic state of stress, which involves depletion of many nutrients. A few months of extra nutrition and avoidance of new stress can restore the body's reserves.

Pregnancies should be spaced — 2 or 3 years is usually adequate — to allow the body to replenish itself with nutrients and new tissue.

Studies have been done of the parents of very outstanding people, and on the average the parents were several years older than the general average. Both social and biological factors are involved. Studies of the biological factors suggest that the optimum age range for the mother is between 27 and 37. In higher social classes, with better environmental support, the average baby is heavier, healthier, and more alert, and has a higher probability of surviving to adulthood; the optimum age increases as income goes up. That is, in Guatemala the safest age for both mother and baby might be 19; in the U.S. ruling class, it might be 39.

On the average, each baby up to the 4th or 5th is bigger and healthier, but then there is a sharp decline in the average; it is at this point — which suggests that reserve nutrients have been depleted — that twinning and Down's syndrome become more likely. The mother's teeth also tend to fall out at that point. Calcium and vitamin B12 are centrally involved in the "apparatus" of cell division. Close spacing of pregnancies, poor nutrition, stress and toxins including alcohol and smoking are all known to increase the rate of birth defects.

Anxiety, as in "schizophrenia," decreases uterine blood flow; it is known that women who become pregnant while they are "schizophrenic" selectively abort the more fragile male embryos. The orgasmic pleasure state is not compatible with anxiety, and would seem to guarantee a better blood (and thus nutrient) supply. Good sexual attitudes probably optimize trans-placental nutrition.

Alcoholic fathers seem to produce as many birth defects as do alcoholic mothers. There are probably other more subtle nutritional effects acting through the father, but so far there isn't much clear information on this.

The mother's brain and the mother's liver both seem to make specific contributions to the baby's nature. Both have profound effects on the ability to make sugar available for the development of an optimum baby. Estrogen is regulated centrally or crucially — by the liver. Estrogen, progesterone, iodine, sugar and stress are closely linked with each other, and with brain development.

Copper and iron can be toxic. Pregnancy and nursing increase all nutritional requirements, with the possible *exception* of vitamin D, copper and iron; it seems to act like vitamin D, improving calcium deposition. Calorie intake should increase slightly (e.g., 200) in pregnancy, and considerably in nursing (e.g., 1000). Zinc, folic acid, B12, and probably B6, and vitamin E; requirements are increased more by pregnancy than by nursing, while protein, other B vitamins, calcium, iodine, and probably magnesium, vitamin A, and possibly fats, are needed in larger amounts for nursing.

IRON SICKNESS

Iron pills and tonics are a big American institution. Doctors often routinely prescribe iron on the same day they determine that a woman is pregnant. Iron pills are known to frequently upset the stomach, but not many people suspect that "morning sickness" could be iron poisoning. The recommended daily allowance of iron for women is about 18 milligrams, but I have seen advertisements in medical journals for pregnancy pills containing several times that dose, without any warning of possible dangers. It is known that excess iron accumulates in the liver, since there is no mechanism for excreting it. It has been noticed that infections, such as malaria, are higher in people who are getting an iron supplement. In tests *in vitro,* iron damages the capacity of antibodies to destroy germs. In the body, iron appears to be "hidden away" during infections, because of this effect on the immune system.

Since iron dosage is so often increased during pregnancy, we should know the scientific background of experiments on animals. All mammals that have been studied need vitamin E in order to get pregnant and to maintain the pregnancy. About 1940, laboratory animals being fed a commercially manufactured diet started showing signs of vitamin E deficiency, dying of softening of the brain. The manufacturers knew they had added vitamin E to the mixture, but when they tested it they found that it contained none at all. It turned out that the iron salts which were added to the food destroyed the vitamin E. The same process can happen in the intestine when iron pills are taken with a normal diet. Natural sources of iron, such as red meat, wheat bran, wheat germ, or molasses, don't seem to have this destructive effect on vitamin E, so if an iron supplement is needed during pregnancy these foods would seem likely to lower the risk of a vitamin E deficiency and of dangers such as a miscarriage.

Iron pills are often used to treat anemia. There are situations in which iron pills could make anemia worse, or even be the cause of it. In a vitamin E deficiency, red blood cells become fragile and break. This type of "hemolytic" anemia is fairly common in premature babies, and is now treated with vitamin E. But anemia is too often treated in adults with the routine iron pills, without considering whether the anemia involves fragility of the red blood cells that might be made worse by iron pills that destroy vitamin E. Old people and cancer victims are known to have abnormally fragile red blood cells. Since estrogen seems to oppose some of the functions of vitamin E, it would seem reasonable to consider the role of vitamin E in anemia, before giving a woman iron pills.

Hypothyroidism is a common cause of anemia, possibly acting through the simple mechanism of lowering body temperature so much that blood production is retarded.

FERTILITY

Avoiding anti-thyroid foods, increasing use of eggs and milk; also, possibly liver with thyroid, progesterone (especially when miscarriage is threatened), magnesium, and vitamin E.

BREASTFEEDING

Several years ago in a biology course we were talking about immunology and I learned that proper American biologists "knew" that the mother's antibodies, though present in milk, were all destroyed by the baby's digestive enzymes, and so couldn't possibly offer the baby any immunity against infections. However, I knew that Romanian scientists, and other unacceptable types had demonstrated that milk antibodies do confer immunity, and that various dietary proteins can enter the body undigested. About 1973, some Americans began discovering that human milk is good for human babies, and helps prevent diseases. It is not going to be so easy now to convince American women that the best nutrition for their babies comes from a "formula," of cow's milk, sugar, and vegetable oil. But foreign babies are still being killed by American companies that dress their saleswomen in nurses' uniforms to convince poor women that their babies need the scientific American "formula," even when there is no clean supply of water to mix it with. Since dietary proteins can get into the blood, early feeding of non-human milk would seem most likely to promote the development of allergies.

Proper development of the face, including the shape of the jaws and alignment of teeth, is promoted by normal nursing, and interfered with when the baby is fed from a bottle. Extensive studies (such as that done recently by J.W. Prescott) show that pleasurable skin stimulation is extremely important for proper psychological development: brutality, rape, religious activity and competition are high in societies which don't give physical affection to infants. Among other animals, even momentary separation following birth damages social behavior. Prescott criticizes bottle feeding, and refers to Aristotle's belief that the state of mind is dependent on the state of the body: "the care of the body ought to precede that of the soul," and "Therefore, the highest good is some sort of pleasure..." (By 1979, human milk is starting to be accepted as the correct food for babies. What is still resisted is allowing the mother and baby to remain in contact, with no separation following birth.)

BRAIN DAMAGE AND THE PUBLIC HEALTH PROTECTORS

Until the late 1950's, boric acid was still in general use as a "safe" antiseptic, and nursing mothers were advised to use it for "cleaning" and "disinfecting" their nipples, so their babies would be protected from germs. Then a columnist reported that some babies had died from getting too much boric acid with their milk, and that smaller doses could cause nerve and brain damage. This publicity discouraged some of the most dangerous uses of boric acid, but the last time I noticed the contents of Listerine mouthwash, boric acid was still included.

In the early 1950s, hexachlorophene started being used by U.S. hospitals to wash newborn babies. Recently, experimenters washed newborn monkeys in the same way, and found that it was being absorbed and was causing gross brain damage. For twenty years, Americans had kept themselves and their children clean-smelling with phisohex and lifebuoy soap, in the belief that hexachlorophene was harmless. How much dyslexia, hyperactivity, and "minimal brain dysfunction" has resulted from such chemical pseudo-cleanliness? Brain damaged animals are known to become aggressive; could poisoning be a cause of human aggressiveness?

A few years ago J. W. Olney of Washington University School of Medicine found that large doses of monosodium glutamate cause brain damage in baby mice, but that the effects aren't obvious until they start to grow up. A typical effect of this kind of brain damage is that the females lose interest in sex and become obese. Since young animals are most susceptible to injury, he criticized the manufacturers who added it to baby foods to make the taste appealing to the mothers who had become accustomed to the taste of MSG or Accent. As a result of the public concern about monosodium glutamate, the baby food companies announced they were no longer adding the substance; instead they quietly substituted another amino acid with a similar flavor. Olney has demonstrated that other amino acids, such as aspartic acid, can be just as poisonous as glutamate. The FDA takes the line that he hasn't proved MSG to be toxic to human babies.

Now the FDA has given its approval to a new chemical sweetener, aspartame, which is a molecule containing aspartic acid. An FDA scientist said, "We do not deny that certain doses of aspartic acid produce brain lesions...' but "Everything has its toxicity: under abnormal conditions, water can be toxic." Stanley Glassner, a consumer-safety officer" in the FDA, expresses his concern in these words: "...on the practical side, I wouldn't say everybody should substitute it in their diets." "Sugar has been around for years, and nobody is dying from it. Any new substance, despite all the safety tests, is surrounded by question marks." Of course, there are many studies that contradict his claim that nobody is dying from sugar, but the most interesting thing is how these men argue, as if sugar or water had anything to do with the subject — we don't want the FDA to regulate sugar and water, so we shouldn't ask them to regulate a fine new product for which consumers will pay a "premium price." The FDA calculated the allowable amount of aspartame on the basis of adult body weight: the allowable amount would have to be smaller if a child's body weight were used as the basis. But the foods that can contain it under the FDA guidelines are foods that children normally eat: sweet breakfast cereals, chewing gum, puddings and gelatine, toppings, and dry bases for drinks, as well as in powder or tablet form. In the form of a "table substitute for sugar," it seems that it would be easy for a child to get a toxic dose.

Since Olney has shown that glutamate and aspartame have an additive effect ("half a dose of each equals a full dose of one alone"), children who ate food containing MSG would have a significant chance of going beyond the so-called "safety margin" for aspartame. The FDA chooses to ignore Olney's clear evidence that these two amino acids have an additive toxicity. Beyond this known menace (though no one knows whether humans are more sensitive or less sensitive than mice to these poisons) there is the possibility of their toxic interaction with other food additives. Food additives are not the "traces of chemicals" many people suppose: for example, nearly half of the calcium contained in commercial bread may come from the dough conditioner and mold inhibitor, with the rest being provided by the milk and wheat. And there are always impurities in the additives, resulting from the industrial processes of their manufacture, but the FDA normally likes to ignore these. When evidence was presented showing that saccharine can cause cancer, the FDA suddenly remembered the impurities in food additives, and now asked for proof that it was "the saccharine itself" that caused cancer, and not an impurity in it. Of course the consumer eats the impurities with the saccharine (and with all other additives), and probably wouldn't care very much whether it was the sweetener itself or the arsenic, mercury and lead in it which caused his cancer. Periodically, women's hair is found to be loaded with arsenic, and the soap companies are told to spend a little more money to remove some of this contaminant, but the pressure of profits always seems to lead them back to the high levels of impurities.

Infant brain damage can be caused by a deficiency of the B vitamin, folic acid. Taking estrogen, as in birth control pills, tends to deplete the body's supply of folic acid, so that if a pregnancy occurs right after stopping the pills it is more likely to lead to a miscarriage or deformity from folic acid deficiency. This vitamin, and probably other nutrients such as zinc and vitamin E, should always be packaged with birth control pills or other forms of estrogen, or at least should be recommended by the doctor who prescribes them. Animal experiments show that giving estrogen to the mother causes brain damage in the fetus. This could result from a folic acid deficiency, or from various other effects of estrogen, such as low blood sugar or high copper.

HYPERACTIVITY

The various tissues of the body can function acceptably at different levels of nutrition. For example, the skin, with its low energy requirements, seems to remain alive for several hours after the death of the body in general. The brain, with its extremely high energy requirements, is usually the first to suffer from energy deprivation. At slight levels of deprivation, the brain will simply lose functional efficiency, but more serious or prolonged deprivation can produce lingering modification, or even structural damage which is relatively permanent (and may even have transgenerational effects.[1])

Just as the skin (or muscle) has a lower energy requirement than the brain, the various parts of the brain have different requirements. The parts which are most resistant to damage are the "lowest" (or "most skin-like") and "oldest" parts of the brain, the parts we have in common with frogs. These parts regulate physiological processes, such as breathing, and so it is biologically useful that they should be most resistant to damage. When a person is given an anesthetic, the first parts to stop functioning, or to go to sleep, seem to be just those parts that have the highest energy requirements, and which are least resistant to damage. The anesthetized person keeps breathing, for example, until very high doses of anesthetic are given, but other functions disappear one by one as the dose increases.

The front part of the brain, which is most uniquely human (and "newest") but which doesn't have "specific" function, in the usual sense, is one of the most sensitive parts of the brain. It is a very large piece of tissue, and it seems to be involved in planning and choosing, in governing the other more specific functions. (This part of the brain, as well as the cerebral cortex in general, gives us the ability to "disregard" stimuli, to use Lendon Smith's term.)

The famous Russian neuro-psychologist, A.R. Luria, has described the behavior of dogs when this tissue is damaged or removed:

> ...destruction of the frontal lobes leads, not so much to a disturbance of memory as to a disturbance of the ability to inhibit orienting reflexes to distracting stimuli...such an animal cannot perform tasks involving delayed responses under ordinary conditions, but can do so provided that irrelevant, distracting stimuli are removed (if the animal is kept in total darkness, if tranquilizers are administered, and so on).
>
> The role of the prefrontal cortex in the synthesis of systems of stimuli and the creation of a ***plan of action*** is manifested not only in relation to currently acting stimuli, but also in the formation of active behavior directed towards the future.[2]

Various theories of what causes hyperactivity, e.g., low blood sugar, weak radiation from fluorescent lights and TV[3] or food additives[4] and the observation that drugs which stimulate the sympathetic or adrenergic nerves (ephedrine or caffeine, e.g.) will relieve the symptoms, all are consistent with the idea that not enough energy is being supplied to permit this tissue to function properly. Low blood sugar will starve the nerves; food additives (which are usually associated with low quality foods with a high sugar content, so this theory isn't nearly so plausible as the idea that eating sugar is the main cause of low blood sugar and the associated hyperactivity) or any low level poison can serve as a stressor of nerve tissue, leading to increased energy requirements; many forms of very weak radiation[5] can lower the efficiency of metabolism, increasing its energy requirement, and brain tissue is the most sensitive tissue to at least some kinds of radiation.

Children who are given amphetamines to keep them quiet in school don't grow as fast as they should, and remain permanently stunted even after stopping the treatment. This kind of drug can be addicting, resulting in decreased alertness when the drug is stopped. Hormonal compensation is likely to be involved, so it would seem reasonable to check at least the thyroid function in children who have been subjected to amphetamine treatment; it might help them catch up in mental and physical growth.

A recent study showed a clear association between small physical defects and hyperactivity implicating "gestational stress," e.g., hormone imbalance and malnutrition, in producing hyperactivity. These could result in either damage to the child's brain or its hormone regulation, e.g., low thyroid and high estrogen. Damaged girls tend to be too passive while boys are too active.

1. Needham, A.E., ***The Growth Process in Animals,*** Van Nostrand, Princeton, N.J., 1964.
2. Luria, A.R., ***The Working Brain,*** Basic Books, N.Y., 1973.
3. Ott, J., ***Health and Light,*** Devin-Adaire, Old Greenwich, Conn., 1973.
4. Feingold, B., ***Why your Child is Hyperactive,*** Random House, N.Y., 1975.
5. Frey, A.H., & S.R. Feld, "***Avoidance by rats of illumination with low power nonionizing electromagnetic energy***", *J. Compar. & Physiological Psychology 89* (2) 183-188, 1975.

FLUORIDE

Water that is naturally "fluoridated" tends to be "hard," that is, rich in calcium and magnesium. A few studies have compared dental health in areas that have hard or soft water, and have found that dental health varied with hardness of water, independently of fluoride content (Rothman, et *al, J. Pub. Health Dent. 32,* 225, 1975; T. Ockerse, *S. African Med. J. 18,* 225, 1944).

Human and animal experiments have shown that good general nutrition, including adequate protein and vitamin C and a high ratio of calcium and magnesium to phosphate, can improve dental health.

Several years ago a study was done to compare blood enzymes in a town before and after fluoridation of the water supply. Changes did occur, showing that the chemical had altered cellular metabolism.

Industrial pollution is tending to raise the fluoride content of soil and water. Foods on the average, in a study done several years ago, contained about ten times as much fluoride as is considered desirable in the water supply. Because of the wide distribution of foods, people in low fluoride areas will still get considerable amounts of it in their food. Burk and Yamouyannis showed an association between fluoridation and cancer, but there seems to have been no discussion of this in the scientific community, other than some distorted comments by the fluoridation establishments.

I think it would be more rational to help people understand the role of nutrition in health, including dental health, than to divert their attention from the real issue (our national food supply) by conducting hysterical campaigns to fluoridate the public water supplies.

"Expect poison from the standing water "

"Those that put their Bodies To endure are Fools."
William Blake

---

6. DIETS

OBESITY

Several years ago, the death of a young physician from blood clots, while she was using a linseed oil supplement, caused me to realize the urgency of getting more information on the toxicity of unsaturated oils into an easily understandable form. While I was writing my dissertation, more than 20 years ago, I saw that there was already abundant research on their toxicity, but commercial propaganda for the "health benefits" of the "good unsaturated oils" (from seeds, nuts, and fish) had caused many people to overlook their harmful effects. At that time, it was clear that they promoted cancer, heart disease, and various degenerative diseases, and even premature aging. Agricultural research had demonstrated that they promoted obesity, and biochemists could demonstrate a specific interference with our most essential respiratory enzymes. Although I knew of experiments in which rats grew fat according to the degree of unsaturation of the fats in their diet, regardless of quantity, and grew lean in proportion to the percentage of (relatively saturated) coconut oil in their diet, again regardless of quantity, I didn't get around to making practical use of these facts until I had spent several months reading the whole history of research on the biological effects of dietary fats.

The idea of "essential fatty acids" (sometimes called "vitamin F") appeared in the 1930s, as a result of tests in which rats developed a skin disease on a fat-free diet, and recovered from the skin disease when fed unsaturated fats. (Other researchers at that time observed that the rats became hypermetabolic on the fat-free diet, as though they were taking thyroid hormone; it was later discovered that the unsaturated fats inhibit the secretion and transport of thyroid hormones, and block the ability of tissues to respond to them.) Shortly after the concept of "essential fatty acids" was proposed, another group recognized the rats' skin disease as the typical changes produced by a vitamin B6 deficiency. They fed rats a fat diet until the symptoms appeared, then cured the disease with a vitamin B6 supplement, without any of the supposedly essential fatty acids. The high metabolic rate of the rats, on a diet without the inhibitory oils, made them eat more, and they needed more vitamins as well as more calories. The high metabolic rate of animals fed coconut oil simply reflects the fact that coconut oil doesn't contain a toxic amount of the anti-thyroid, anti-respiratory unsaturated fatty acids.

Americans have a lower metabolic rate than some other cultures, and the result is that obesity is a major problem in this country. Since farmers had demonstrated that coconut oil (though it is cheap) was not good for fattening their animals--it made them lean and hungry--and since cancer researchers showed it could lower the incidence of cancer, I began adding it to my diet. At first I noticed that I felt warmer after eating it, as if I had taken a thyroid supplement. Then I noticed that I was losing weight, while eating more calories than normal, because of adding about an ounce of coconut oil to my usual diet. After several months, I leveled off at a weight about 15 pounds lower than my "normal" weight of the previous 26 years. As some of my friends learned what I was doing, they began eating coconut oil, with the same results. The biochemical basis seems clear: The easily oxidized short and medium-chain saturated fatty acids of coconut oil provide a source of energy that protects our tissues against the toxic inhibitory effects of the unsaturated fatty acids, and reduces their anti-thyroid effects. The animal studies of the last 60 years suggest that these effects also provide protection against cancer, heart disease, and premature aging. Other effects that can be expected include protection against excessive blood clotting, protection of the fetal brain, protection against various stress-induced problems including epilepsy, and some degree of protection against sun-damage of the skin.

While the use of coconut oil makes it possible to go longer without eating, because its pro-thyroid effect increases the liver's ability to store glycogen, frequent snacks are still important for helping to lose weight, or to prevent weight-gain. The mechanism is partly that smaller meals cause less insulin to be secreted, and insulin turns on the fat storage process, and increases appetite. Another important mechanism is that the liver provides about 70% of our active thyroid hormone, by converting thyroxine to T3, but it can provide this active hormone only when it has adequate glucose. Frequent snacks--for example, sipping a few ounces of orange juice about every hour— keeps the T3 level up by providing glucose to the liver. (Snacks shouldn't consist of protein by itself, since protein stimulates insulin, but not T3, secretion.)

APPETITE

Low blood sugar usually causes an intense craving for something sweet. It is known that a vitamin A deficiency causes increased hunger — I suspect this acts through the mechanism of blood sugar. A deficiency of vitamin B1 causes loss of appetite. Normally, appetite is probably a good indicator of specific needs for protein, fat, carbohydrate, vitamin C, salts, and possibly other nutrients. As our tastes evolved, they had to be satisfied by whole foods, so a craving for carbohydrate wouldn't disrupt our physiology if we didn't have such easy access to highly purified (or distorted) carbohydrates.

A craving for "salt" is normally satisfied with sodium chloride (in bacon, cheese, crackers, olives, etc.), which doesn't meet the body's needs. Taking sodium as an additive suppresses the hormone which enables the body to retain sodium, and so it is physiologically addictive. In addition, the precursor hormone may accumulate, and this hormone produces inflammation (in joints, especially, as shown by the work of Hans Selye and his associates). If we could satisfy the salt craving with a balanced salt, including potassium and magnesium and calcium, we would probably be more comfortable and would avoid the salt (sodium) addiction. Low thyroid can cause loss of appetite. Thin people, even very active people, can still be deficient in thyroid.

FASTING

The thymus gland, essential for immunity, shrinks during fasting. Chronic infections such as tuberculosis are more common in malnourished people. However, fasting has been used successfully in treating certain diseases. It can be useful in diagnosing food allergies, as in some types of schizophrenia. Its use as a weight reducing technique is probably not generally justified by the facts. A current study (1975) is investigating the possibility that a balanced salt solution will prevent the destruction of muscle and other protein-rich tissues during fasting. I have noticed that such a solution relieves feelings of stress, so I think it will prove to prevent protein-wastage.

In a study of the nature of weight loss in a two week fast, it was found that about 95% of the lost weight was from protein rich tissues (muscles and glands), rather than fat. A low calorie diet produces a slower weight loss, but in this case most of the lost weight is fat. Since fat has a very low rate of metabolism, people who lose muscle by fasting are going to have increasing difficulty in losing weight, since they will have less active tissue to consume fat. Building up muscle and lymph tissue for optimum health — even if it initially causes a slight weight gain — will make reducing easier by increasing the mass of metabolically active tissue. Progesterone is the only steroid hormone I know of which will cause the thymus to regenerate. Vitamin A spares protein, and will protect these tissues even on a fairly low protein diet (Vits & Hormones, 1977).

Chronic dieters can adapt to a low calorie intake (Lancet, April 5, 1975, Miller and Parsonage). This is probably partly from a loss of active "protein tissue." Total nutrition is needed for replacing such tissues.

Fasting and stress suppress the thyroid, and thus can aggravate many symptoms. Thyroid function isn't always restored when the fast ends.

COFFEE, TEA, AND COLAS

Coffee, cocoa, and cola are flavorings made from seeds, and tea of course is an extract made from certain leaves. This means that they must contain nutrients as well as drugs. This fact — that an extract made from plant or animal tissue contains nutrients — is very commonly overlooked. Even the companies that sell the products incorrectly describe them as containing no nutrients, except the other materials they add to the flavoring. For example, Coca-Cola claims that phosphoric acid and sugar are the only nutrients in their product, yet a standard text book indicates that Coke is rich in potassium (while Pepsi has more sodium than potassium). In a study of the thiamine content of dark roast coffee, it was found that one or two cups provide the minimum daily requirement of vitamin B1. Leaves contain magnesium, potassium, vitamins A, K, E and Q10 (ubiquinone), as well as other trace minerals and the B vitamins, so all kinds of tea must contain moderate amounts of these nutrients. About 20% of dietary niacin and manganese can be provided by coffee. In Russia, green tea is often prescribed for its vitamin P or rutin content. Seeds and leaves often contain chemicals which bind materials such as magnesium, zinc, and calcium, but these will break down and release the minerals under various conditions — the fermenting process in tea manufacture, for example, should have this effect.

Some nutritionists have noticed that caffeine is said to raise insulin levels in the blood, and from this have reasoned that, since insulin promotes the conversion of glucose to fat, caffeine must be avoided in a reducing diet. Caffeine has a reputation for raising blood pressure, but the evidence is not clear on this point: it seems to be an individual matter whether it will raise or lower blood pressure. Caffeine, in fact, is prescribed in doses equivalent to 2 to 4 cups of coffee (200 to 400 mg.) to relieve hypertensive headaches (J.P. Merrill, in *Principles of Internal Medicine,* Harrison, 2nd edition, p. 1425). Coffee improves circulation to the brain; Benjamin Franklin and Goethe are said to have used 30 to 65 cups daily. This amount would be close to the maximum safe daily dosage of caffeine, 6 grams (Bennett and Bondy, *Principles of Internal Medicine,* p. 795). Very small doses of caffeine have a "paradoxical" sedative effect, but this is a familiar effect of anything which raises the brain's energy level.

Caffeine (which doesn't necessarily have the same physiological effect as coffee) stimulates the sympathetic nervous system and raises the cellular level of cyclic AMP. Both of these effects promote lipolysis, the removal of fat from storage for use. This may account for the fact that coffee has been found to lower serum cholesterol and triglycerides, while raising the level of free fatty acids. Increased lipolysis would seem to be desirable in connection with a reducing diet. (Incidentally, estrogen *lowers* the level of cyclic AMP in most tissues.) Since both caffeine and adrenalin raise the metabolic rate, fat is presumably being consumed more rapidly. Adrenalin is known to raise blood sugar, apparently by inhibiting the utilization of glucose and increasing the utilization of fat. Coffee normally raises blood sugar, by its adrenalin-like effect. In this case, the level of insulin doesn't seem to be the primary factor regulating carbohydrate metabolism. However, during fasting, coffee and/or adrenalin might speed the depletion of the glycogen reserves and thus speed the appearance of hypoglycemia. Many of these studies seem to indicate that coffee would be a valuable part of a reducing diet, but since the results are so contrary to "common knowledge," there will have to be more experimental work done. Other factors, such as the habit of sweetening coffee, also have to be considered. An interesting study in the USSR suggests how complex these experiments can get: animals were fed either boiled water or unboiled water, and it was found that the animals receiving boiled water had significantly higher serum cholesterol levels than the animals drinking unboiled water.

Caffeine, acting through nerves as well as directly, can increase immunity. Injected into an animal's brain, it was found to slow the growth of cancer. It was recently discovered accidentally that a very small amount of caffeine mixed with the tars from cigarette smoke prevented that material from causing cancers. It was also found, in an experiment with cultured cells, that caffeine prevents the multiplication of a cancer causing virus. Caffeine stimulates the thyroid, and hypothyroidism can cause extreme susceptibility to infection. Epidemiological studies show that heavy coffee drinkers have no more heart disease (or other sickness) than non-drinkers. However black women seemed to be protected against heart attacks if they drank coffee.

Still, coffee makes many people anxious and can produce a stress-like reaction. Whether to use it or not is largely an individual matter.

NATURAL VITAMINS AND MINERALS — ANY DIFFERENCE?

Most biological molecules are produced in only one of two "mirror image" forms. Even natural (e.g., "right-handed" or "left-handed") chemicals can be degraded by harsh industrial processes into a more random mixture. The structural randomization is called racemizing. An interesting theory of aging is that racemic molecules accumulate with time; these molecules are known to have different physical and biological properties. Synthetic vitamin E may be cheap and easy to standardize, but the randomness may also be responsible for the slight toxicity of high dosages of vitamin E reported by a few doctors.

The idea that "an element" such as potassium is simply that element, without further qualification, is a strange idea to be proposed by anyone who supposedly has had a chemistry course, but that is what the American Dietetic Association says. Elements come in different isotopes; the proportion of heavy and light isotopes of, for example, potassium, varies in the human body with age, and is measurably different from normal in cancer cells. "Natural" minerals are usually bound by special molecules, such as proteins or "pigments" (e.g., heme) and in this state do not seem to destroy vitamins, as do various water-soluble "inorganic" minerals. Chelation does not necessarily improve assimilation of a mineral — in fact it often *prevents* absorption of a nutrient, as in the case of phytic acid.

The A.D.A. officials who propagate nutritional misinformation may be honestly ignorant, or they may think it is in the public interest to lie. Either way, it is quite wrong for them to so aggressively attack the "nutritional quacks" when their own information is so dubious.

ADDITIVES AND QUALITY

An American Dietetic Association "Position Paper" on food and nutrition misinformation says "Judicious use of food additives helps ensure high quality processed food." That may in some warped way be true, but it has nothing to do with the reality of food manufacturing. A reference book on additives for the food industry points out that you shouldn't *always* buy the lowest quality cheap food materials, and then attempt to give them the appearance and flavor of higher grade food by the manipulation of chemical additives, because sometimes the necessary additives are so expensive that it might occasionally be more profitable to buy a better grade of food material in the first place. This agency, when talking to the food industry, is perfectly frank in acknowledging that additives are used for the purpose of foisting inferior grades of food upon the gullible consumer. Why is the A.D.A. so intent on denying the facts? (If an apologist for the A.D.A. reads this: consider it a challenge to a public debate on the subject of your choice.)

A study was done about 30 years ago to see whether supplements given to "exceedingly well-nourished" tuberculosis patients would make a difference in their recovery. The supplement consisted of 600 milligrams of vitamin C, 75.000 to 150,000 units of vitamin A, 5000 units of vitamin D, about 4 grams of brewer's yeast, and six grams of dried liver. The control group received placebos, in "double blind" fashion. There was a distinct improvement in the group which got the supplement (see Williams' *Nutrition Against Disease,* p. 223). So many similar studies have been done it is simply unscientific to say that supplements aren't necessary when "well balanced" meals are eaten. At a symposium for pharmacists, the "professional dietitians" were arguing that druggists should not sell any nutritional supplements without a prescription. A woman in the audience pointed out that most Americans don't take the time to prepare three "well balanced" meals every day, and that they just won't be well-nourished if they don't take some kind of supplement. The dietitian snickered "I am defeated," but went on with her plea that the druggists stop selling supplements, with the strong implication that she couldn't argue with such irrational opponents.

Individual peculiarities and stress can make it extremely difficult to stay healthy on a normal diet; however, if meals of liver, broccoli leaves and oysters and papaya can be considered normal, then supplements might generally be unnecessary.

If a person develops symptoms of hay fever, a chronic cold, asthma, diarrhea, hemorrhoids, headaches, numb fingers, dizziness, etc., it is possible that they are allergic to some of the trash which is used in the manufacture of the pills; powdered vitamins and minerals might be tried in that case, since they are more likely to be "pure" — but even these powders can contain allergens. See "Warning About Supplements." Low blood sugar, as shown by H. Laborit, will induce allergic reactions even when there was no sensitivity at a higher level of blood sugar. Since low thyroid is an important cause of low blood sugar, thyroid function should be checked (by BMR or achilles tendon reflex, even by body temperature, but not by blood tests) when there are signs of allergy.

WARNING ABOUT SUPPLEMENTS

As we age, we accumulate more and more of the heavy metals in our tissues. Lead replaces calcium, and it reaches concentrations in the bones many times higher than in the soft tissues. A bone meal supplement produced at a glue factory (where the animals were probably old) was found to contain 190 parts lead per million. The FDA has set a limit of 1½ part per million for evaporated milk, but they refused to act in the bone meal case in 1970 because they said food supplements were in a "gray area" between food and drugs; they now say they recognize health foods as food. More recently, a survey of dog food found over 5 ppm lead, again probably because of the age of the animals used. Fluoride also accumulates with age in bones. The lead in our bones is less harmful than the same amount in our soft tissues, but certain materials (chelators, including penicillamine and EDTA; bottled salad dressing often contains EDTA) are able to remove lead from bones and move it to the brain, where it is more destructive.

Another supplement that is likely to be dangerous is "lecithin," in the form usually sold. Lecithin itself is white. When exposed to oxygen the unsaturated fatty acids oxidize, causing it to become yellow and then brown. Rancid oils are dangerous — see pages 117-118. Eggs are a good way to get fresh lecithin. Use of a choline supplement will stimulate lecithin synthesis in the body when the essential fatty acids are present. Whole foods (leaves, seeds, etc.) are less likely to have deteriorated from exposure to oxygen than are manufactured foods.

It is hard to separate cadmium from zinc, and cadmium is toxic, so zinc supplements should be used carefully. Biological purification (as in oysters) is usually more effective than industrial refining.

The FDA has allowed some very strange uses of the word "natural" — in their sense, industrial processes are natural. Vitamins E, A, and sometimes D are available as natural, biological substances, but other vitamins are not. Tablets often contain paraffin and talc (which contains asbestos fibers) as the supposedly "inert" binders.

VITAMIN C: MANY EFFECTS

One of the oldest known functions of vitamin C is its role (hydroxylation) in the synthesis of collagen for connective tissue. At high concentrations, it can also depolymerize (make more soluble) the collagen, reversing one of the important features of the aging process. A recent study (J. Clin. Nutr. summer, 1974) shows that even inside the cells of membranes structural integrity is improved (electron microscopic evidence in guinea pigs) by very high doses, including the large doses suggested by Linus Pauling. Since infections have to enter through membranes, structural integrity would seem likely to improve resistance. Tyrosine metabolism, which is involved in brain function, is sensitive to vitamin C; also, vitamin C maintains tissue adrenaline levels, possibly by inhibiting its oxidation, and adrenaline is necessary for the chalones to exert their function of inhibiting cell division. (Pauling proposed a role for vitamin C in controlling cell division in cancer, but the mechanism he chose probably wasn't the correct one; there may be a variety of mechanisms, including for example the free radical processes suggested by W.F. Koch and A. Szent-Gyorgyi.) Hans Selye has demonstrated that vitamin C can prevent heavy metal (e.g., mercury) toxicity; it reduces the metal to a less toxic form, and also helps solubilize and remove it. White blood cells have an extremely high affinity for vitamin C, and can't function properly without an adequate amount: because of this great affinity, an excess of white cells, as in leukemia, apparently robs other tissues of vitamin C and produces hemorrhages and bruises.

Some people oppose the idea that nutrition can prevent or cure diseases. Many strange warnings about vitamin C have appeared in the newspapers.

INTERACTIONS

Since all nutrients work together, it's generally best to eat a variety of foods at each meal. Unrefined foods assure a fairly broad range of nutrients. People sometimes forget that meat is a "refined" food in this sense: it doesn't contain all the nutrients needed to make an animal. Nearly all Americans have porous, weakened bones and teeth by the time they are 50, because of the large amount of meat eaten in relation to other foods. When excess phosphate (from meat or wheat germ, for example) is eaten, calcium and magnesium are removed from the teeth and bones to be excreted with the phosphate. Using a large amount of milk improves the ratio of calcium to phosphorus, but doesn't supply enough magnesium to prevent tooth decay, heart trouble, and cramps. Greens and vegetables should be eaten with the animal proteins.

Eating extra amounts of liquid oil will increase your need for vitamin E, and extra carbohydrate will make you need more vitamin B1. Excess protein increases the amount of B6 needed. Some kinds of protein (cysteine rich, such as muscle and liver) also inhibit the thyroid; carbohydrate can promote the formation of T3, the most active form of thyroid hormone.

Other types of interaction haven't been very well studied, but they probably are the reason for some peculiar diet systems: allergies to one food can cause digestive problems that interfere with other foods. For example, people who are allergic to onions sometimes have a gall bladder reaction which prevents proper digestion of fats. If we added up all of the special "avoidance" diets, no one could eat anything. Many people are ruining their health by avoiding too many foods.

CEREALS, SEEDS, AND BEANS

A seed is a kind of storage device, usually containing enough material to produce a sprout and root several times bigger than the seed, just by adding water. Health food "fanatics" for many years have advocated the use of sprouted grains and beans, and used to be ridiculed by the scientific home-economist types who "knew" that a seed contained all the nutrients that would be in the sprout. Home economists did approve of soaking beans overnight, but only because it was supposed to reduce cooking time. E. Pfeiffer used to demonstrate chromatographically how very different sprouts were from seeds in chemical composition, but it is just in the last few months that establishment (Colorado State University) food chemists have reported that sprouts contain twice as much protein as do the legumes from which they grow.

Glutin, the main protein of gluten, is a typical storage protein. Instead of the normal ratio of nitrogen to carbon, oxygen and hydrogen, glutin is extra heavily loaded with nitrogen, in the form of amide and amine groups on the side chains. When seeds are soaked or sprouted, these nitrogens combine with carbohydrates to form a large amount of new protein, consuming in the process some of the stored starch. If we eat seeds in the crude form, our digestive enzymes handle the glutin differently, producing some fairly toxic peptides (chemically related to histamine) and some ammonia; these, added to the starch, can cause gas and a variety of allergic reactions. Phosphate is also released from its storage form as phytic acid by sprouting. This reaction also produces inositol, to which the phosphate is bound. If seeds, especially legumes, are eaten without soaking, phytic acid chelates minerals such as zinc and prevents their absorption. The traditional practice of letting bread rise overnight allowed these same enzymic reactions to occur. The hasty baker is not only robbing the population of half of its cereal protein, but is also making a slightly toxic product. (Thyroid inhibitors — iodate and bromate — are added to most bakery breads.)

VINEGAR, HONEY, AND FAT

I have seen people very quickly get fat on a daily drink of cider vinegar and honey and a dose of lecithin. The folk medicine tradition behind it was probably valid — it was a good way to fatten up people who were under-weight. But somehow this got twisted into promoting it as a "reducing formula." Lecithin is a good nutrient and seems to lower the danger of a high cholesterol level in the blood. And cider vinegar and honey are both rich in necessary minerals. But the acetic acid in vinegar not only is a component of fat molecules, but it also serves to activate the process of converting glucose into fat *(Adv. Lipid Res.* 9, p. 111. 1971). Thus the formula is good as part of a weight-gaining diet, but not as part of a reducing program.

MARGARINE OR BUTTER

Animal studies show that margarine causes more circulatory disease than does butter or cholesterol. Margarine is produced from oils (which may be rancid) by the use of a nickel catalyst; a trace of nickel remaining in the oil could be harmful, but it is probably the synthetic form of fat itself which is toxic. This is another case where a synthetic chemical is entirely different, biologically and chemically, from the natural chemicals. Hardening at best would cause the oil to become like animal fats (hydrogenated), but reality is worse than theory, and hardened oil is worse than animal grease. Butter has other valuable components, including vitamin A, while margarine often is colored with very dubious dyes — nutritious carotene used to be used, but now synthetic mineral dyes are usually more "economical." (I don't know whether this is still true — Aug. 21, 1979.)

LIQUID OILS

E. Racker and other biochemists have pointed out that the unsaturated (liquid) fatty acids are able to uncouple the energy producing reactions from oxidation. This means that they will promote consumption of fuel without increasing fat synthesis. This is an effect similar to the "specific dynamic action" of proteins, and it is the biochemical explanation for the fact that all calories don't count the same as far as weight reduction goes. But this also means that all useful energy production is reduced in relation to heat production.

The unsaturated oils also can stimulate a dangerous kind of oxidation, in which they break down in ways that seem to accelerate the aging process. One of the more conservative investigators of vitamin E recently (in *A.J. Clin. Nutr.,* 1974) revised his opinion regarding the required amount of vitamin E: he wrote that the requirement of 15 mg./day will be increased to about 50 mg./day if the person eats much unsaturated oil (fish, seeds, etc.). People who study the amount of vitamin E needed for reproduction, and those who study its effect on the durability of red blood cells usually come up with very different figures for an optimum intake. The age of the animal or person studied is crucial: in the first year of life, the minimum dose for fertility in rats increases by 67 times. The only study of vitamin E needs in human menopause that I know of suggest that 500 mg./day is needed.

Extrapolation of the rat results to humans would suggest a little bit more than that.

A study comparing Dutch babies with English babies found that the amount of unsaturated fat in the body was about 40 times higher in the Dutch babies who were fed very little animal fat. The vitamin E requirement increases as the amount of unsaturated fat in the tissue increases.

In a big study to test the idea that liquid oil would help prevent heart disease through its effect of lowering blood cholesterol levels, the raw figures showed slightly more heart disease among the liquid fat eaters, though the difference wasn't statistically significant. There was, however, a significantly greater rate of death from cancer among the liquid fat eaters. An animal study done about 1940 suggested that this would happen: animals fed large amounts of cod liver oil nearly all died of cancer, but when they were fed the same amount of oil with a large vitamin E supplement, their cancer rate was normal. It's startling to realize that the whole group conducting the experiment failed to anticipate this result, through ignorance of the literature on animal studies of liquid oil feeding.

Some articles in medical magazines have claimed recently that an effect of diet on heart disease has been demonstrated, but they neglect to point out that the dieters also stopped smoking — and the known effects of smoking would account for the differences in heart disease.

Since unsaturated fats poison energy production, they could even contribute to heart disease. They inhibit thyroid function, and hypothyroidism is associated strongly with heart disease. In a recent study, people who ate large amounts of unsaturated oils were judged to be older in appearance than people who ate less.

Recent studies are showing that animal fats (saturated) are essential for proper brain development, and that unsaturated fats (as in typical "formulas") can damage brain development.

LAXATIVES

The daily use of a few spoonfuls of bran in the breakfast cereal, or of a carrot as a snack (or grated, as a salad), can prevent practically all constipation. A high fiber diet also lowers the risk of bowel cancer, and is being used increasingly for preventing and treating conditions such as colitis and diverticulitis. It turns out that the popular old "bland diet" without fiber was just about the worst possible thing for colitis. An extra benefit of carrot fiber, besides the bulk and moisture-holding properties, is that it captures and holds fat molecules, removing them from the body and making weight loss easier. The small amount of sugar in carrots is released slowly, so that it doesn't disturb blood sugar as much as would the same amount in a different form.

It is now known that even "purified" mineral oil contains small amounts of cancer causing chemicals. Mineral oil isn't just a benign lubricant, it is an irritant. Years ago, autopsies of chronic users of mineral oil found that the oil had entered fat tissues, where it stayed because it can't be metabolized. When "authorities" say that mineral oil can't be absorbed by the body, I wonder what kind of a mechanism they have in mind that would keep it out while other oils are being massively absorbed.

If a person really needs a laxative, one with fewer dangers would be preferable — maybe Epsom salts or aloe vera. Chronic constipation is a very common sign of hypothyroidism. Premenstrual constipation, gas and diarrhea are also associated with low progesterone.

SPECIFIC DYNAMIC ACTION

Stillman's diet book is one of the few contemporary publications to mention the fact that "specific dynamic action" of proteins leads to a variable fattening effect for a given number of calories. This is a good point in an otherwise poor book, and it is in direct contradiction to a popular establishment argument, that "a calorie is a calorie," and that weight loss is possible only by cutting calories or exercising. "Increased energy expenditure" is misleading, because the specific dynamic action of proteins (and of unsaturated fatty acids) increases energy expenditure without changing overt activity.

The idea that "a calorie is a calorie," or a simple calorie counting approach fails to recognize not only the specific dynamic action of proteins (the action of oils is usually called "uncoupling of oxidative phosphorylation"), but also fails to recognize events at the organismic level, such as insulin secretion, which form a link between the form in which food is taken (composition and timing) and the behavior, appetite, and metabolism. For example, an active brain can burn about half of all the energy consumed by the body. If brain activity is depressed, a very large percentage of the food consumed becomes available for making fat. Most physicians, who should be in the habit of considering the person as a whole, will still tell you that a "calorie is a calorie." The fact is that for many people, 100 calories of sugar is profoundly different from 100 calories of protein, even when both are taken as excess food beyond an adequate diet. The sugar will affect not only the way it is used, but it will modify the body so that the other food is not used properly.

Avoiding stimulation of the insulin-secreting beta cells in the pancreas will tend to make energy more continuously available for normal functions, including mental alertness, instead of storing it as fat. This amounts to a kind of "systemic dynamic action." Diets which take advantage of this principle are Atkins' low carbohydrate diet, and Gordon's "Wisconsin" diet which involves frequent small meals and a fairly high protein intake. The type of protein is important, since some kinds suppress the thyroid and slow metabolism when used chronically in large amounts.

Sometimes eating more protein will increase heat production, but this can't happen unless the thyroid is working fairly well.

HCG

Many reducing clinics are using injections of the pregnancy hormone, Human Chorionic Gonadotrophin, for the purpose of making reducing diets easier and possibly improving fat distribution. This hormone shifts energy metabolism toward the use of fat rather than sugar, and so allows the blood sugar level to rise. This suppresses appetite. The hormone is produced by the placenta to make sugar available for the growing fetus. It helps the placenta to develop fully, and has been shown to have a profound influence on the development of the brain of the fetus. HCG and similar hormones produce more intelligent offspring both in animals and humans.

A suppressed or "quack" method of diagnosing for cancer has been to use a "pregnancy" test on the urine of the patient (Beard Anthrone Test), because it was believed that the same metabolic shift occurs in both cancer and pregnancy. It is now recognized by normal scientists that cancers produce *many* peptide hormones, frequently including HCG, so the pregnancy test should sometimes work as a cancer test, though it probably isn't reliable.

Recently, Dr. G.G. Costa and others at the Medical College of Virginia developed a test for cancer which probably involves this "pregnancy metabolism." They feed the patient some radioactive fat, and a person with even a very small cancer will breathe out about three times as much radioactive carbon dioxide, showing that the metabolism shifts toward fat mobilization at an early stage of cancerization.

Cancers, like embryos, live mostly on sugar. High blood sugar is maintained by causing the body to consume itself (fat and protein) while leaving sugar for the growing tissue.

HCG is very important for the health and intelligence of babies. It certainly should make reducing easier, but at present it seems risky, since it could promote the growth of a hidden cancer. Until it can be shown that this doesn't occur, I think HCG should be used only during pregnancy, when it is helpful in strengthening the placenta. Some cancers are caused to grow faster by pregnancy, and HCG might have the same effect. However, it might also turn out to help in treating some kinds of hypoglycemia. It shouldn't be suppressed mindlessly, but neither should it be promoted mindlessly.

NOTE FOR DIETERS

While it is true that the hypothetical "well balanced meal" can provide adequate nutrition for most people, you should remember that part of that concept, well balanced," is the assumption that the total intake will be big enough to supply the "proper" amount of calories, usually between 2,000 and 3,000 per day. The three areas in the world with the greatest life span have a normal diet of about 1200-1900 calories per day. Although standard texts still claim that 1600 calories a day is the minimum for maintaining body weight, recent studies showed that some women can't lose even on 1000 calories a day. The attitude generally has been that if a woman doesn't lose weight on 1200 calories per day she must be cheating. A "normal" diet has to be, among other things, one which doesn't produce destructive obesity. But have the advocates of the unsupplemented well balanced diet studied the proportion of the Recommended Daily Allowance in a 1200 calorie diet? Until the question has been studied properly, it isn't scientific to oppose supplements or special foods. Many Americans, especially women, deliberately restrict their food intake, so this is a question of general concern.

POPULAR REDUCING DIETS

First, the worst: Dr. Stillman's "inches off diet" is low in protein and designed to cause muscles to atrophy. This tends to make a person flabby, shapeless, and weak. By shrinking active tissue, it makes it easier to put on fat, and harder to use it up. His other diet, low in carbohydrate, is the same as Atkins'. The A.M.A. has been warning about the dangers of this "ketogenic" diet, and of course it could be dangerous to a diabetic who takes insulin and then eats no carbohydrate. But both sides of the argument were presented in *Medical Counterpoint,* and Dr. Atkins cited several dozen appropriate scientific publications to support his position. The man supporting the A.M.A.'s position found about half a dozen references to cite — one of them was a textbook documenting his quotation of the first law of thermodynamics. Maybe there is a valid reason for opposing this diet even under a doctor's supervision, but if there is, the A.M.A. hasn't demonstrated that it knows what it is. The Eskimos who used to live on meat and fat all winter seem to have proven that people can tolerate such a diet.

Many dietitians insist that you must have at least 100 grams of carbohydrate daily because the brain "uses glucose." However, the brain can adapt to using the ketones which result from fat oxidation.

Gordon's "Wisconsin" diet provides about 40 grams of carbohydrate with 90 grams of protein in a daily diet of about 1250 calories, and so is making use of the principle of low carbohydrate intake, though to a moderate degree which most doctors find acceptable — especially since there is a strict limitation on calories. The most interesting part of Gordon's diet is that the day's food is divided into at least six meals, or three meals and three snacks. This procedure is based on experiments with animals, in which the rats that learned to eat their daily ration all in one meal got fatter and fatter, while rats that ate the same amount, but could nibble on it whenever they wanted, didn't get fatter. In the wild state, this would be useful, since it would mean that when the animal found food it could store a large part of it as fat, to use later when food was scarce. But when food is always available, instead of getting fat the nibbler feels more energetic and spends the energy in activity. I have worked for a company (Medical Diet Service, in Portland and Seattle) that has kept records on thousands of people using the Wisconsin diet, and the system seems very effective. Counseling and "portion controlled" packaging of food are part of the program there, but a motivated person could get similar results, weighing their portions on a food scale and avoiding all refined carbohydrates. Getting some protein, carbohydrate and fat in each meal or snack seems desirable for many hypoglycemics, but often changes have to be made such as increasing the calories and eating more often. Diabetics sometimes use the same diet.

I have seen publicity about something called the NASA astronauts' diet, and was impressed by the large amount of refined sugar in it. One of the newspaper stories about it included a picture of a broken-down astronaut. I'm not sure what the purpose of the diet is, but I wouldn't advise a friend to eat it.

People talk about the "Mayo diet" — I think it consists of grapefruit and bacon — but the Mayo Clinic regularly denies any connection with it. I don't advise anyone to eat commercial bacon, because of the nitrite which is added to it. The nitrite combines with amino acids to make a type of chemical, the nitrosamines, which are known to be powerful cancer inducing agents. The chemicals appear in dangerous concentrations if "preserved" meats are left at room temperature for a few hours. The smoke used in bacon, ham and sausages is also suspected of causing cancer. And the amount of salt in bacon would probably cause retention of water (temporarily; most people adjust quickly to altered salt intake). Otherwise, the "Mayo diet" probably works for some people who can't lose weight because of their craving for carbohydrates, and are too lazy to learn a little about nutrition. It would eventually cause cramps, tooth decay and softening of the bones because of the small amount of calcium and magnesium.

DIET PILLS

Amphetamines mimic the action of the "alarm" part of the nervous system (sympathetic) and so raise the level of blood sugar; this is probably the mechanism (or part of it) which suppresses appetite. Low blood sugar is associated with hyperactivity, and this is probably why the same drug is effective for the hundreds of thousands of crazy kids who get it so they will sit still in school; coffee works as well in hyperactivity, and might also help dieters. Another drink, desert tea or squaw tea (ephedra) is also effective. Coffee, unlike other stimulants, activates the thyroid gland.

However, a recent study found that in a group of 100 patients with Hodgkin's disease, 19 of them had previously used amphetamines, while only three out of 100 matched controls used them. This is apparently another effect of mimicking stress, or forcing the blood sugar up. Tonsillectomies have also been associated with an increased rate of Hodgkin's disease. Stress damages lymphoid tissue, and tonsils are composed of this tissue; Hodgkin's disease affects the same kind of tissue.

It has been found that diet pills are only temporarily effective, and when discontinued the fat returns.

FAT: IDEAS FOR GETTING OFF A PLATEAU

Fiber, such as two raw carrots per day. Coffee, as a trial, when there aren't reasons against it. Avoiding cabbages (unless cooked), mustard, radishes. Try going off estrogen treatment — usually, natural progesterone works better for controlling menopause symptoms, is less toxic, and stimulates the conversion of food to heat and energy, and use of stored fat. Vitamin' A and pantothenic acid promote natural progesterone synthesis. Iodine, manganese, and cobalt are all possible problems in thyroid functioning. Related to hormones and blood sugar, get the liver healthy, for example by eating liver at least twice a week, etc. Consider allergens, like onions, etc., that could be disturbing the liver. Sleeping less will help keep blood sugar up and fat down, unless the brain is really tired. Lower room temperature and brighter lights will stimulate the thyroid. If acne or dandruff occur, a vitamin A deficiency is suggested. Vitamin B12 and vitamin E are both needed to make use of vitamin A efficiently. Gelatin helps keep the blood sugar up, by stimulating glucagon release, and so helps control hunger. Medium chain fatty acids, found in coconut oil, are effective in turning off fat synthesis in the liver.

ONE WOMAN'S TYPICAL DIET FOR A DAY

Soon after waking, a piece of fruit. For breakfast, an egg and cereal or toast (using pre-soaked grain for the cereal or bread); milk on cereal, butter on toast. Two hours after breakfast, a snack of cheese (1/2 ounce) and raw carrot. For lunch, a tuna salad; fruit or milk, if more calories are needed. For supper, maybe oyster stew and a salad and a potato — or, a chicken breast, well boiled spinach or broccoli, and fruit. Just before bed, another snack of milk and fruit.

SWELLING UP (EDEMA)

Proteins are very large molecules, which don't pass very easily through the walls of blood vessels — and if they do leak out of the blood vessels into the space around cells, there are enzymes there that can dissolve them. So the blood stream maintains a high concentration of proteins, normally, which by osmosis tends to make water enter the blood from the space around the tissue cells. These proteins are largely produced by the liver. If the liver isn't functioning well, or if there is general stress, or if there isn't enough protein in the diet, these proteins tend to disappear, with the result that water accumulates outside the blood vessels. In the morning, this water will be visible as puffiness in the face, especially under the eyes, but by evening gravity will have moved it to the feet and ankles.

Not enough protein and too much sodium are the most common causes of edema. High estrogen just before menstruation often causes it. Estrogen promotes retention of sodium, which in turn helps the body to hold water. Myxedema, which results from insufficient thyroid hormone. involves leakage of proteins out of the blood vessels, and apparently a shortage of the enzymes which should dissolve them. High estrogen blocks various proteolytic enzymes, apparently including those which release thyroxine from the colloid in the thyroid gland since it causes colloid to accumulate (colloid goiter) while reducing hormone release. It also antagonizes the actions of thyroxine on tissues. Besides eating adequate protein, it is necessary to have adequate vitamin A and zinc for efficient protein synthesis. Vitamin C and rutin (grapefruit is a good source) are needed to maintain integrity of blood vessel walls. Other nutrients are needed for normal liver functioning.

Chronic edema contributes to premature wrinkling and other signs of aging.

Members of the cabbage family (including radishes, mustard, broccoli and cauliflower) contain a chemical that interferes with thyroid function; cooking reduces this effect. Peanuts and soybeans can also interfere with thyroid function, but they act in the intestine, preventing absorption of iodine, so their effect could be overcome by eating a little extra iodine. These or similar antithyroid materials in various foods apparently account for the existence of goiters and cretinism in some areas where the soil contains a normal amount of iodine. The absence of other nutrients, such as cobalt, can contribute to the development of goiters.

EXERCISE

In the 1950's a national survey revealed that physical competence in the US had deteriorated, but it took J. F. Kennedy's example to make exercise popular. While jogging became popular for preventing heart disease, we were frequently told by experts how many miles a person has to run to burn off a pound of fat. However, in Russia, physiologists always remember to include the brain in their calculations, and it turns out that a walk through interesting and pleasant surroundings consumes more energy than does harder but more boring exercise. An active brain consumes a tremendous amount of fuel.

In the last century, Sechenov found that exercising one hand strengthens not only that hand, but also the other. Brain activity stimulates growth and alteration of tissues, such as the muscles. Once I decided to attend a modern dance class which began the next week. After two or three days of visualizing myself in unusual postures and movements, my muscles started feeling the way they do the day after a long hike, though I hadn't actually done any exercise. This effect of nerves on other tissues is called their trophic effect: it actually changes the chemical composition of muscle, its weight, and other properties. In the US, yoga is usually thought of either as a system of exercises, or as a strange sort of religious practice. However, at least some of the Hindu yogic traditions considered visualization to be the point of the exercise, and recognized that the body could be powerfully influenced by mental activity. Recently psychologists have claimed that attention and visualization can cause breasts to enlarge. Even sensory nerves (such as the pain sensing nerves in the cornea of the eye) have a powerful trophic influence — so maybe it isn't just a myth about massage being useful in reducing. Bright lights also stimulate hormone production and energy metabolism, and increase muscle tone.

Many dietitians claim that exercise doesn't increase the need for protein, but the Russians have found that a combination of exercise and increased protein intake can increase the muscle mass. In a woman, this process can not only improve grace and body proportions, but it also increases the body's ability to burn up fat. Other nutrients are needed for using protein properly, and for maintaining optimum nerve functioning. However, if the exercise produces too much stress and not enough muscle action, muscles will atrophy as a result of cortisone's shifting amino acid metabolism into glucose production. Lactic acid production (getting out of breath) is the main signal of the need to produce new glucose. Therefore, "aerobic" exercise is the most stressful. Cortisone not only causes atrophy of skin, muscles and immune system, but it even has been found to accelerate aging changes in the brain.

Stress uses progesterone and can cause menstrual periods to stop. Girls who begin regular exercise (such as dancing) before puberty have later sexual development.

Exercise increases blood clotting, and so can *increase* the risk of strokes and heart attacks. Some doctors have been reporting increased incidence of flat feet, varicose veins, and prolapsed uterus among joggers. Walking is a better form of exercise.

ONE MEGAVITAMIN PROGRAM

Each person has unique nutritional requirements, and these will vary under different circumstances, but here is a program that some people use during stress. Ninety grams a day of protein, preferably including liver, eggs, milk and seafoods. Fruits and starchy vegetables can make up the rest of the calories. Calcium and magnesium, 1200 mg. each, potassium chloride 2 to 4 grams, zinc 20 to 30 mg., iodine about a fifth of a milligram, and manganese and other trace minerals from seafoods, such as kelp. Vitamin B1, 5 to 20 mg. Vitamin B2, 20 to 30 mg., Niacin, 100 to 500 mg., with the requirement sometimes increasing just before menstruation. Vitamin B6, 10 to 50 mg. Pantothenic acid, 100 to 500 mg. Folic acid from 1 to 5 mg. Biotin, 1 mg. Vitamin B12, 25 to 100 micrograms (100 micrograms is the same as one tenth milligram). Inositol and choline, about 500 mg. each. Vitamin A, 50,000 to 100,000 units, always taken with vitamin E (200 to 400 units of d-alpha tocopherol). Rutin and the bioflavonoids are sometimes used when capillaries are abnormally fragile (some types of purpura, petechial hemorrhages, and spontaneous bruising have this cause). Vitamin D from fish liver oil, up to 2000 units a day in winter unless pregnant. The evidence for vitamin D toxicity is based on the synthetic form of the vitamin, but remember that vitamins A and D (and other oils) can be toxic in large amounts. It's interesting to compare the official propaganda about vitamin toxicity with the official silence about many of the dangers of drugs and food additives. A few major medical and pharmaceutical crimes are documented in the book *200,000,000 Guinea Pigs.* In the U.S., vitamin K is available only by prescription, but is contained in leaves. In the U.S.S.R., vitamin B15 is recognized and used, but in the U.S. it is utterly banned: the man who discovered it insulted the A.M.A. The same man also studied laetrile (I-mandelonitriles), sometimes called vitamin B17, which is suppressed as a cancer therapy, but is a common substance that is available in many seeds, such as grains and apricot seeds. There has been a great campaign of lies against this material, including stories (even on a TV doctor program) that two or three apricot seeds can be lethal.

Potassium chloride should not be used by anyone with bad kidney function, since it could accumulate, slowing or even stopping the heart. It should not be taken in tablet form, since a high local concentration stops intestinal movement, leaving the tablet in one spot where it can burn and cause ulceration. A potassium chloride powder (such as Morton's salt substitute, which is not contaminated with ammonium chloride) can be sprinkled on the food. It is best to get your potassium from foods, such as fruit.

ADAPTING TO A NEW DIET

Enzymes are continually being destroyed and synthesized in active tissues. When a vitamin binds to its enzyme, it helps to stabilize the enzyme against degradation, leading to a higher concentration of the enzyme. In the same way, the "substrate" of an enzyme (the material it changes chemically) can stabilize the enzyme. When we eat a diet that is very low in a particular nutrient, such as protein, we lose many of the enzymes involved in handling that nutrient. Without those enzymes, a meal rich in protein, for example, can liberate more ammonia than the body can dispose of, and the person can be poisoned. Many vegetarians have experienced this "toxic" effect of meat or cheese or milk, and so believe that "animal foods" can cause mental dullness. headaches, dizziness, etc. But for a meat eater, the same process can cause vegetables to produce gas, as slow carbohydrate digestion lets bacteria break them down. Changing to any new diet, or ending a fast, should be done gradually, allowing at least several days for enzyme adaptation. The same rule would probably apply to nutritional supplements. If gas is a problem even when change of diet isn't responsible, a thyroid deficiency should be considered. Lack of stomach acid is typical in hypothyroidism, but is only one aspect of a generalized digestive depression.

ENERGY ITSELF: CrP and ATP

Although electronic energy is intimately involved in life, there are two chemicals that are involved in maintaining the "energy charge" of cells, and it is the energy charge which is most immediately related to biological function and structure. Creatine phosphate (CrP) is a kind of energy reservoir for muscle, and in a vitamin E deficiency creatine leaks out of the muscles. Aging also seems to involve defective creatine phosphate reserves (Verzar). Adenosine triphosphate (ATP) is more directly involved in all kinds of life function, for example maintaining the resting state of nerves and muscles, and governing secretion, the retention of proteins, and the elimination of toxins. ATP is more stable than many chemists realize — it is only a lack of magnesium or an excess of calcium which destabilizes its molecular structure. This seems to be involved in the sedative and anti-cramp actions of magnesium. Sensory nerves can release ATP into surrounding tissues, and this seems to be part of their "trophic" influence on healing and inflammation. A.E. Needham *(Growth Process of Animals)* has discussed the possibility that it is a "vitamin": when added to the diet of animals, it increases their growth. This must have some relevance to our nutrition, since fresh food contains abundant ATP. A day or so after an animal dies, "rigor mortis" develops because of the disappearance of ATP; a similar loss of ATP occurs in plants as they die. For many decades, fresh food enthusiasts have spoken of the "life energy" in fresh foods. Unfortunately, most scientists and health professionals still like to mystify the subject and deny that food could contain "vital energy," or that ATP could have nutritional significance.

GENERAL PRINCIPLES OF GOOD NUTRITION

1. Minimize your requirements by avoiding unnecessary stress. In Oregon in the winter, use *bright* lights, balancing incandescent bulbs with fluorescent tubes.

2. Avoid toxins. Run water 1 minute before using, and then only from the cold faucet. Do not cook tomatoes or fruit in iron or copper pans. Don't use pewter dishes. Avoid mineral oil and other solvents on skin or in air (most cosmetics contain mineral oil, and worse). Minimize contact with allergens. Be very careful with unsaturated oils, such as safflower, corn, and cod-liver oil: they destroy vitamin E and can cause cancer. The "heart diet" is a menace based on

weird professional ignorance. These oils interfere with the thyroid gland.

3. Grains, legumes, and some nuts (e.g., walnuts and peanuts) are highly allergenic. Soaking or sprouting them is very desirable. Cooking cabbage, broccoli, cauliflower, mustard, etc., will destroy chemicals which poison the thyroid gland. Laetrile and PABA inhibit the thyroid. Greens and potatoes (cooked) are good to substitute for bread (especially the factory-made kinds) and for beans. Soy beans are terribly over-rated.

4. Eat frequently, using protein, fat, and carbohydrate at the same time, e.g., an egg and an orange, or a carrot with cheese. Fruit is the best source of carbohydrate; avoid uncooked starches such as nuts.

5. Use complex foods, things close to their living state: eggs, sardines, leaves, milk, etc.

6. Heat degrades protein. Canned or powdered milk has lost significant amounts of lysine, an important component of protein. The same applies to toasted cereals, nuts or beans. The heated lysine forms a carcinogen if a sugar is present, as in soybeans.

7. Any drug alters your nutritional needs. Tobacco, iron, aspirin, estrogen, tranquilizers and diuretics must be taken into account. There are special diets for special needs.

8. Don't get a "diagnosis" from anyone but a physician or other licensed person. But don't think that diagnosis is so scientific that you take an individual's opinion as the last word. For example, a girl had wasted away to 90 pounds and thought she would soon die from "pituitary atrophy," but switching from raw foods to milk and eggs allowed her to regain her weight. Diagnoses also sometimes label a serious condition as something less serious. The appropriateness of

any diet will depend on the accuracy with which your nutritional needs are known.

9. Besides their content of the essential nutrients, all natural foods contain other materials, such as hormones. There are many nutrients which are useful, without being "essential" in the narrowest sense. Under some conditions, nutrients which are not normally essential may become so. Nutrients that are synthesized by intestinal bacteria must be taken in the diet when antibiotics are used.

10. If supplements are necessary, don't use them excessively — find what is enough, but don't forget the contaminants and adulterants which may be present in pills, capsules and powders. Amino acids such as tryptophan or glutamic acid should not be used as isolated supplements.

11. A few years ago, most of the nutritional problems that I saw were caused by physicians, by refined convenience foods, and by poverty. Recently, most of the problems seem to be caused by badly designed vegetarian diets, or by acceptance of the idea that 40 grams of protein per day is sufficient. The liver and other organs deteriorate rapidly on low-protein diets. Observe the faces of the wheat-grass promoters, the millet-eaters, the "anti-mucus" dieters, and other low-protein people. Do they look old for their age?

12. Everyone should know the basic principles of nutritional physiology and have a general idea of the chemical composition of foods. Otherwise, you will be confused by conflicting claims. Become your own expert — for example, if someone tells you not to eat fruits and proteins at the same meal, get a book on digestion and absorption of food from the library, and read about interactions.

13. Examine your basic assumptions about food and life and health, and those of the experts. Is the organism a rigidly determined genetic mechanism? Is it the sum of its past environments? Does it really assimilate the environment? Is it a desire for more life? What is pleasure? Is a person a spirit temporarily trapped in a large piece of meat? Scientific questions often take on a clearer meaning when you can see their ideological context.

14. If someone who claims to be an authority belongs to a "professional organization," look at the publications of that organization. What were they advocating 5 or 10 years ago? Are there financial motives behind their recommendations? Be suspicious, keep asking questions.

7. THE FUTURE

HIDDEN MOTIVES

When scientific or professional publications are financed or controlled by special financial interests, we should watch for distorted reasoning, distortion by selection, and plain misstatement of facts. The Nutrition Foundation, Inc., is an important source of nutritional information in the U.S. Their trustees include officers (presidents, vice presidents, chairmen of boards, chief executives) of these companies: Coca-Cola, Royal Crown Cola, Oscar Mayer, Miles Laboratories, Hoffmann-LaRoche, Proctor & Gamble, Kellogg, Philadelphia Macaroni, Stauffer Chemical, Skinner Macaroni, Specialty Chemicals Group of ICI United States, and Dobbs-Life Savers. Can we expect their publications to be properly critical of synthetic food additives and highly refined foods?

DISESTABLISH THE PROFESSIONS

We hear a lot about the "controlled scientific studies" that supposedly have to be done before anyone can advocate something as risky as taking a nutritional supplement. The controlled nutritional studies that have been done always seem to have the wrong national origin, or have been published in "obscure journals," so that they can be ignored. I want to point out that many of these criticisms are incompetent not only because of what they ignore or suppress, but because of their double standard: if the scientific standards they demand of nutritional studies are applied to medicine, we have to say that there is no "adequate scientific basis" for many of the practices of modern medicine. Tradition is extremely important in the practice of medicine. Consider the common appendectomy or tonsillectomy. Are these practices based on animal experimentation? On human experimentation?

What animal disease would be comparable to appendicitis? Would human experimentation require the sham surgery which is a standard requirement in scientific animal studies? Sham surgery would require that people in the control group with appendicitis be cut open, without removing the appendix. Since the stress of surgery can actually affect the immune system and various physiological processes, controlled studies would not be entirely unreasonable. What other therapies have been compared with surgery in treating tonsillitis and appendicitis? If you have seen the old horror movie, "Freaks," or if you went to a circus side show in the 1940's, you can visualize the effects of an operation called a "hemicorporectomy" that was favored about 35 years ago as a treatment for a cancer of the lower part of the body — it involved removal of the lower half of the body. What kind of "controlled scientific study" was this based on? The establishment has committed itself to extremely rigorous scientific standards in its attack on nutritional therapies — and there is an extremely large body of nutritional research which meets these standards. We are therefore perfectly justified in demanding that the food, drug, and medical industries meet the same rigorous standards. (Since I wrote the above, there have been some studies of tonsillectomy and appendectomy. For example, acute appendicitis usually does not require surgery, according to the latest study.)

A PROPOSED STUDY

Many of the well publicized specialists in misinformation say that it is impossible for human beings to be deficient in vitamin E, and so we mustn't try to draw any conclusions about human sterility or miscarriages from the animal studies which showed that vitamin E is essential for implanting the embryo and maintaining pregnancy. Technically, this is known as Pig Ignorant Professionalism. The chemical processes in food don't care whether the food is consumed by rats or by people. When iron salts are added to food which contains vitamin E, the vitamin E is destroyed by the iron. When pregnant women are given pills containing up to 2000 per cent of the daily iron requirement, this iron mixes with food. The amount of money that is spent on propaganda against vitamin E could support some simple little studies to determine whether inorganic iron supplements increase the risk of miscarriage. This would seem to be a reasonable concern — is there equivalent evidence to justify the campaign against vitamin E? I don't think so.

PROTEIN AND STARVATION

At first glance, proteins seem to be required in human nutrition, in fairly large amounts. Many people are dying of what is called a protein deficiency, or a combination of protein and calorie deficiencies.

But a Russian found that atmospheric nitrogen was incorporated into body proteins by higher animals. It had been thought that only certain bacteria (such as live in the roots of legumes) could fix atmospheric nitrogen, turning it into ammonia for use in amino acids and proteins.

Then an Australian group studied New Guinea highlanders who lived on sweet potatoes and bananas, and found they excreted vastly more nitrogen than they ate, yet they remained healthy. They guessed that nitrogen fixing bacteria lived in their intestines. It turned out that E. coli, which lives in everyone's intestine, gives the chemical reaction indicating nitrogen fixation.

Then a group in Illinois (Dudka et al., Nature 232, 265, 1971) found that the amount of atmospheric nitrogen breathed in was not the same as the amount breathed out.

What is essential seems to be the "carbon skeleton" of the essential amino acids. If the diet supplies these along with other nutrients, then protein seems to be not so essential in the diet. If fruits and vegetables can be found which contain these substances, then the world food problem could be easily solved. Why aren't starchy, sugary and oily plants (including bananas and sweet potatoes) being surveyed to find a source of these nutrients? Since this special problem isn't "my field," I couldn't hope to get government financing for such a study. But someone should be doing it. (The protein quality of potatoes is higher, according to animal feeding experiments, than it should be, according to amino acid analysis. One of my students has demonstrated the presence of these. "amino acid equivalents" in potatoes.)

REASONING ABOUT HEALTH

"What is now proved was once only imagin'd"
William Blake

The famous logician, C.S. Peirce, said that a kind of tying-together, or "colligation," of "a variety of separately observed facts" is a "generally essential step in reasoning." This process is too often excluded from formal scientific reasoning.

Tying together, forming chains of probable relationship, perceiving a cluster or constellation — these are a necessary part of any productive scientific work. In working toward a scientific goal, such a perceived constellation or pattern will direct experimentation which attempts to fill in some of the blanks in the pattern. If certain blanks remain empty, it may be necessary to re-draw the road map leading to your goal. Sometimes a person will claim to have reached a certain goal using a strange new kind of road map; if the goal is important, it's worth seeing whether the new map is a reliable way to reach the goal. Magazines like *Prevention* are full of articles using this sort of goal-centered reasoning; there is nothing in the history of science to indicate that this isn't a valid way to proceed. However, there are some Establishment slogans that are being used in an effort to suppress any dissenting opinions in medicine and nutrition. "Raising false hopes" is one such slogan, as if being respectably sick meant abandoning all hope; but allowing the patient who stays under "proper medical care" to hope for a miracle seems perfectly acceptable.

DIETETICS OR NUTRITION?

"Always be ready to speak your mind, and a base man will avoid you."
William Blake

Dr. Andrew Weil recently mentioned that, after getting his medical education at Harvard, he doesn't recommend going to doctors. He says "preventive medicine" is a phrase everyone uses, but doctors get no training in what it means — for example, he said his training in nutrition consisted of a half hour lecture by a dietitian describing what diets were available at the hospital. Other medical schools give twice as much training in nutrition as Harvard, but even in a whole hour the doctor is likely to learn nothing more than that nutrition is a very simple matter of choosing the right menu from the list provided by a dietitian, and that "a normal balanced diet provides all the nutrients the body can use." On the basis of a 30 minute talk by a dietitian, the "Harvard educated physician" becomes an authority on nutrition (and everything else related to health, though their training has been mainly in sickness, not health), and his "professional opinion" is taken seriously by public and lawmakers.

Since a 30 minute talk by a dietitian is given such tremendous weight in our culture and laws, we should know something about their training: such awesome power, if not divine, must come from the next highest authority, but since that seems to be the AMA, this would involve a circularity.

Dietetics is often combined with home economics. It is still possible to become a dietitian without taking a single course in biochemistry. It isn't too surprising that the textbooks used in their nutrition courses contain little more than is in junior high Health texts. But it is odd that they criticize people with training in biochemistry (e.g., Linus Pauling, Adelle Davis, R.J. Williams) as not being qualified to talk about nutrition. According to a Registered Dietitian whose lecture preceded mine on a symposium for pharmacists, physiologists aren't qualified to talk about nutrition either, and "every quack in the country is calling himself a nutritionist." A friend of mine who visited the Oregon State University nutrition department told me that a display there included books by these people (mentioned above) in a display on "nutritional quacks." Adelle Davis had a degree in dietetics and nutrition, from the University of California at Berkeley, and a master's degree in biochemistry from the USC School of Medicine. Williams, a professor of biochemistry (and the only biochemist to have been chosen as president of the American Chemical Society) has done research in nutrition for over 50 years, and is the discoverer of the B vitamin pantothenic acid, and did basic work on other B vitamins. Pauling, Nobel laureate in chemistry (as well as in peace), created much of the scientific foundation for modern medicine, physiological chemistry, and nutrition. Maybe someone is trying to glorify quackery by associating these people with the word? In judging comments about Linus Pauling, we should remember that U.S. scientists almost ostracized him when he got the Nobel Prize for peace, when war and nuclear testing were part of the respectable American Way. He was not allowed to travel abroad in the early 1950's, and this probably prevented him from getting another Nobel Prize for work with DNA. Many U.S. scientists who hated him for supporting peace now choose to call him a quack.

A study found that people with more education are more likely to eat "health foods." However, a study done by Oregon State University nutritionists found that food faddists' diets are no better than a normal diet (I don't know what they mean by normal; the US Department of Agriculture found that close to half of the US population has a nutritional deficiency, so normal is bad). The dietitian reporting the study on TV said that faddists avoid many of the good foods like white bread, and that we should follow a normal diet to "eat all the food God gave us."

NUTRITION AND CONSCIOUSNESS

"Worldly revolt of the individual comes from an interior revolt that has sought out health and natural physical processes subtle and gross."

Michael McClure

"...the conscious subject has for his object the infinity of his own nature."
"One is what he eats."

Ludwig Feuerbach

"One food (agricultural) scientist is worth more than all the economists in the world."

Karl Marx

There are attitudes, ideologies, and institutions which hate anything that threatens to be useful. Effective knowledge is likely to upset everything that's neatly formalized, including the livelihood of the middle class. Commenting on the hostility of Freudian psychiatrists toward nutritional therapy for neuroses, Aldous Huxley said "poor fellows; what will become of them?" The anthropologist M. Harris says "Sometimes I think that the primary function of establishment anthropology is to fog the truth...It stays away from questions about the causes of war, the causes of sexism, the causes of racism. It stays away from all statements of causality...Academics are the high priests of the inward turning consciousness that has spread through America."

Nutritional knowledge threatens to be useful. Biochemically trained people like Linus Pauling, Roger Williams, Adelle Davis and Abram Hoffer who write about nutrition are called "quacks" by establishment dietitians who may be trained in home economics, and who may not understand, for example, how an iron pill might cause anemia.

Mystification of food takes many forms. I remember seeing in Mexico a horribly poor (i.e. probable daily income less than 20 US cents) woman feeding her baby Pepsi Cola and pieces of a white wheat roll. Those things are heavily advertised in Mexico, and even to people who can't read they represent "class." The institution of eating three meals a day and dessert after supper is a mystification of food. Trimming the fat off your meat and avoiding pork to "keep your cholesterol down" is a multiple mystification.

Honest ignorance exists, but there is also deliberate falsification: consider the claim that additives are used so that we can have high quality food. A publication intended for industrial food chemists tells the story more bluntly, warning the manufacturer that it isn't *always* the best policy to buy the lowest grade of food and then make it palatable with additives, because sometimes the adulterants cost more than is saved. In other words, profit is the only important factor, and sometimes, conceivably, it *might* be profitable to sell good food.

When you start looking for ulterior motives, you might conclude that your physician is greedy, that your chemistry professor has a contract with the rubber company that makes ice cream, and that food producers are so pleased with their profits that they don't care about the increasing numbers of deformed and mentally retarded babies, or the increasing rate of cancer and diabetes. If you do this, then you are probably involved in a demystification of the world. Eating good food can alter your consciousness; so can thinking about how we're going to get it.

ABOUT FEELINGS

About 1959, I realized that feelings of love and anxiety had particular forms and locations in the front of the body. Gradually, I learned that these could be modified intentionally, and that social feelings and senses of personality and place consisted of "conformations" of these plexuses. Even in brief social encounters (of a few seconds), these body feelings may take on a conformation of openness and love, of sexual feeling, or of a closed anxious coldness. In the pleasant experience, the visceral feeling resembles channels which open and extend outward toward the other person; at times, these channels seem to make powerful contact with the other person's. Occasionally, when I feel very energetic, especially on sunny days, I have an intense sensation of sweetness that seems to travel up from behind and below my navel, to a spot behind my sternum. I call this my body's smile energy, because it feels the same as the pleasure which goes with a smile.

When I described these perceptions to an older person, she reported having lost those feelings in middle age, and she said it seemed that they had been "insulated" by the extra fat she had put on. (People who don't notice those sensations may wonder how a person could feel insulated from something which is inside oneself. The point is that they are sensations of openness of the body to the world.) Her comments caused me to associate the feelings with thyroid function and metabolic rate. I have noticed that when I feel sluggish from bad weather or diet, those feelings seem muffled, or barely perceptible.

Recently, I described these body feelings to a friend (in her early twenties) who wasn't sure what I meant. For several weeks, she didn't experience anything that seemed like my descriptions. She began taking thyroid a few weeks ago. Within a few days of the time that she had increased her dosage (from $^1/2$ to 1 grain), she told me that she had begun to feel things she had never felt before, feelings of openness and intensity in her body. Another friend, the same age, said she had orgasms easily when she was 18 and 19, but in the last 2 or 3 years had been unable to. She claimed to have no emotional feelings in her body, even when she desires, except for vibration when she is sexually excited, and an awareness of something in her pelvis. When I mentioned the association between thyroid and nerve reflexes, she recalled that she had been put on a large dose of thyroid hormone in her late teens, just about the time she discovered she could have orgasms. Moving to Oregon, her new doctor had taken her entirely off thyroid. She stopped having orgasms, and begin to have frequent suicidal depressions. A little thyroid stopped her depressions, without increasing her pulse, which was only 60. She consistently increased her use of thyroid, and has since reported having orgasms.

Athletic training is known to slow the pulse. Cortisone, produced by stress, inhibits the thyroid gland. (When the thyroid is low, less oxygen is needed, so this is a useful adaptation for increasing endurance.) These hormonal changes are now known to produce sterility in both men and women. Estrogen, used for birth control, also elevates cortisone and interferes with thyroxine. Estrogen, like a thyroid deficiency, can lower sexual responsiveness. My guess is that heavy exercise, such as running, will lower sexual responsiveness as it lowers fertility. Emotional stress, by causing the same hormonal changes, would have the same effects. Nutritional deficiencies and environmental toxins, by causing stress and hormone imbalance, could do the same.

If someone has never experienced a full sexual response, it is meaningless to ask about the occurrence of "orgasms." Ease or difficulty in responding sexually, though, and perceptions of bodily emotions, might serve as a subtle indicator of hormone balance, especially thyroid sufficiency.

DESIRE, THE LIBERATOR OF SEXUAL OBJECTS

Men, out of touch with their energies and natural desires and dreams, have kept women in chains. Passive and weak, women have kept to themselves the wholeness and richness of their experience.

Reasoning and competing men have believed that they possessed women, but the centered and prolific human female world was overlooked by the greedy devouring male, who took part of her existence and believed he had taken it all.

Wishing to be liberated, no longer passive and weak, many women are becoming reasoning competitors, but in doing so are losing contact with their bodily energies, desires, and dreams.

It is obviously hard to desire the kind of man who has produced, and been produced by, western civilization. He is the competitive athlete or the competitive sedentary business-man, or the competitive intellectual rationalizing his superiority over all beings.

Sexual desire has been so closely involved with enslavement, many women feel very concretely that desire must be overcome if they are to gain full human status. Being a sexual object has meant being enslaved and diminished.

Gaining the social, economic, cultural, intellectual, and sexual rights of men will not liberate anyone, because these rights and roles are where the ugliness of maleness is. It is not the penis that is fascistic, domineering, exploitive, corrupting. The penis is the male animal-flower, a soft-firm dildo, a warm dream.

All objects are desirable, no object enslaves; imposed systems enslave.

If we see that to be an animal, to be human, is to desire, then we see that to be understood is to be understood as desire. If our perception is purified, there is no mere object.

In a society which considers a corporation to be a person, we have to be careful when we ask to be treated as "a person, not an object." The society's definition of a person is something like "an emptiness with rights." We want equal rights, but we also want equal fullness. To achieve that human fullness, men have to be freed from their abstract reasoning aggressive possessiveness, and women have to be freed from their passivity.

Intersubjectivity is possible when we recognize a mutual desire for growth. This kind of contact expands our self and our known world, while allowing the other to expand.

Men relate by looking at the world together. Men and women relate by seeing each other as perspectives on the world. A sexual subjectivity, rather than a sexual object. Intense relationships between women are just beginning to be explored. Intense relationships between men and women should be further explored — new selves will be evolved, and new methods for exploring will be discovered. But before this is possible for everyone, the whole system of capitalist imperialism has to be changed, so that being human is not defined primarily as having an economic role.

Men and women have real differences, but the nature of these differences still has to be investigated, in the course of mutually supported growth.

FERTILE PAIRING

The sexual pair is the unit of invention.

It's as though the brain of each were incomplete. Undoubtedly culture exaggerates some biological differences, but it seems to erect barriers to the kind of interaction that leads to dreaming discovery. Change and adventure are important for our energy system, and the present authoritarian culture is opposed to fundamental change.

In terms of hemispheric balance, girls depart less radically from bilateral symmetry, and reach a mature stability somewhat earlier. This is consistent with their characteristic "global" consciousness, as opposed to the male's analytic style; culture is definitely a factor in shaping these styles, but the larger brain/body weight ratio of the female is likely to be involved — that is, more brain would tend to achieve better balance.

At first, this feminine brain superiority, if we generalize from the general mammalian meaning of the brain/body weight ratio, seems to be a put-down of men. However, the view I am proposing attributes some virtue to the masculine imbalance itself.

When I noticed a similarity of feeling between excited, dreaming, tottering mental exploration and the plain hungry low blood-sugar state, I realized that a certain kind of alertness is like a falling away from old habits.

In this view, masculine consciousness would be characterized as impatiently stumbling along into new territory, while the female provides the understanding necessary for steering an intelligent course.

More creative individuals of either sex probably experience both of these tendencies, cyclically, to a greater degree than does an individual who remains deeply imbedded in the culture, but real mental intercourse of the sexes seems to offer the greatest support for creativity.

From "EVOLUTION AS HUMAN SCULPTURE," 1967

. . . we can begin to think of ourselves, our bodies, as objects, without the old perverse connotations of "possession," "non-living," "passive-mechanical." We can recognize that in changing our viewpoints, we are changing our bodies in real structural ways, and that in spite of the magical nature of our functioning, there are real bodily inertias that we have to work with.

Wanting to complexify our body structures, so that the inertias will interfere as little as possible with the activity of our consciousness, we will use a sort of "material dialectic." When everything seems to be perfectly under control, and is going smoothly, and not much is being learned, it means that we are structurally complex enough for the demands of the situation, and that below the surface of experience there are inertia structures that are slowing our multiplication of viewpoints.

This means that to evolve, and to expand our consciousness, it's time to look for the most improbable, the most demanding, confusing, even threatening, situation. The feeling of adventure that directs the choice of activities is the same as that of a sculptor, thinking and imposing intentions as far as possible, but finding new intentions and new problems in the act of physically attacking the stone with the hands and arms, and in the constant discovery of essential and accidental properties of the stone. We have to believe that there is something really new and important to be discovered.

The redundant torpor of jazz, and the patterned gestures of most dancing are the opposite of adventure, and these things assert that past and present are sufficient, that pleasures are not formative.

The sculptural feeling for the massiveness and resistance of your own body in confronting reality is involved in the sexual process, which is another dimension of evolution. For the active consciousness, perception is emotion; desire is inherent in the perception of a mate, and perception of self is part of the perception of other. For the old consciousness, therefore, desirable characteristics were generally not related to evolutionary values, since the self had only the dimmest awareness of such values. A woman's need for security, in a society which makes women dependent, will cause her to be attracted by wealth and power, without reference to her subtler needs.

Experience is stored in our tissues, and is passed on, but not as Darwinian "gemmules." What is stored is flexibility, potential, and energy capacity. The mate who can challenge by complementary perceptions arouses deep energetic processes, felt as desire, and as knowledge projecting itself into the future. The hormonal and probably electrical changes, the subtle structural changes that appear as increased stickiness, hysteresis, are part of the individual's organismic development, but they are also at the heart of evolution of the species. Great loves make great people. By recognizing, knowing, responding to, more of the other, we evolve the organ of response, the brain.

If this stuff is true, then reproduction should be delayed until there is maximum capacity for response, and a maximum of personal ripeness, to elicit such intense and general responses from a mate.

APPENDIX

Factors in Steroid Synthesis

LDL Cholesterol

Thyroid/Vitamin A

↓

Conversion Blockers: | **Conversion Promoters:**

Mitochondrion

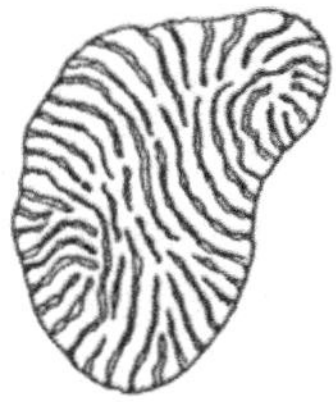

Conversion Blockers	Conversion Promoters
Estrogen	Thyroid
X-Rays	Light
Ultraviolet	Vitamin A
PUFA ("EFA")	Vitamin E
Iron	Copper

↓

Pregnenolone

↙ ↘

DHEA **Progesterone**

Estrogen **Testosterone** **Cortisol** **Aldosterone**

Structural integrity of the mitochondria is essential for functional respiration and steroid synthesis. Coconut oil, thyroid hormone, pregnenolone, and progesterone stabilize mitochondrial structure.

ISOPRENE (Precursor, shows up in nocturnal breath, probably indicating interference with its use.)
CHOLESTEROL (Vitamin A, thyroid, and mitochondria integrity, which depend on factors that limit lipid peroxidation, are needed for its conversion into pregnenolone.)
PREGNENOLONE (Formed in mitochondria, probably exits from that structure by a solubility gradient as well as specific mechanisms, to the cytoplasm, where tissue-specific enzymes in microsomes oxidize it further to either:)
DHEA or PROGESTERONE (These and pregnenolone should be abundant, probably saturating cells to the solubility limit)
ESTROGEN, TESTOSTERONE, CORTISOL, AND ALDOSTERONE (These are the "terminal" steroids, which vary greatly according to circumstances; in excess they are toxic, and in the absence of saturating amounts of the precursor steroids--which are slightly antagonistic "buffers"--even normal amounts can have exaggerated effects.)

The accumulation of cholesterol clearly indicates the failure to convert it to steroids, so elevated cholesterol is a fairly reliable diagnostic indicator of hypothyroidism. The appearance of isoprene in some people's breath during the night is probably an indicator of something interfering with the synthesis of cholesterol. Highly allergic people often have extremely low cholesterol, making it impossible for them to synthesis normal amounts of the protective steroids.

SOME DEFINITIONS

Carbohydrate: a molecule containing carbon, oxygen, and hydrogen, e.g., sugars and starches. The formula is, roughly, any multiple of HCOH.

Collagen and connective tissue: one of the best known "pure" proteins, gelatin, is made by boiling animal skin or other tough tissue to extract collagen ("glue source") which is the main protein component of animals. It forms a tough jelly in which cells are embedded. Other macromolecules, especially hyaluronic acid and chondroitin sulfate, are major components of other extra-cellular materials, such as joint fluid, eye jelly, cartilage, tendons, etc. Gelatin lacks essential amino acids (cysteine, tryptophan) and so nutritionally will not serve as a protein source for general use.

Dietetics: (see Nutrition).

Glycolysis: the degradation of glucose (or glycogen) to pyruvic acid, with the production of a small amount of energy (ATP), relative to the very efficient oxidative production of ATP which consumes pyruvic (or lactic) acid, or fat (or acetic acid) or carbohydrates derived from amino acids. Alcohol not only is oxidized as a "fat," but it apparently inhibits the wasteful conversion of protein to fuel and so allows protein to be used more efficiently. The wasteful glycolysis of cancer can sometimes be controlled by such "physiological" means.

Lipids or fats: molecules containing mainly carbon and hydrogen, though biological fats typically have a carbon oxygen-oxygen group at the end, which increases their solubility in water. These relatively soluble fats are the fatty acids, which can combine with glycerin to form triglycerides (three fats, one glycerin). We synthesize many fats, but some others must be included in the diet — essential fatty acids, or "vitamin F."

Lipolysis: the breaking down of fats, it commonly refers to the breakdown of storage triglycerides into fatty acids and glycerol.

Minerals: generally, these are all the elements that are needed by organisms, but which can be found in nature independently, though carbon, nitrogen, and water are not called minerals. They have structural, chemical, and catalytic functions.

Mitochondria: small "compartments" in the cytoplasm (the viscous part of the cell, everything but the nucleus), they are responsible for much of the cell's energy production (as ATP) and oxygen consumption.

Nutrition: a branch of biology or physiology, an area of scientific study which overlaps many other areas, including biochemistry, physiological chemistry, reproduction and growth, microbiology, general and comparative physiology. etc. Easily distinguished from dietetics, which tends to be concerned more narrowly with the regulation of food intake, but also with cooking and food prices, serving food, and professionalism.

Proteins: with water, proteins are the main structural components of the animal body. They are also the catalysts (enzymes) which govern the rate of almost every chemical reaction in the organism. The third type of protein is used for immunity: antibodies. Proteins are synthesized in cells in a linear manner, connecting many (50 to a few hundred) amino acids in a row, but the most soluble (hydrophilic, water-loving) normally take on a compact, roughly spherical form. They are classed as "macromolecules," molecules which are so large that they have special properties; it is sometimes more useful to think of them as a "system" than as a unit. When proteins are digested, they are broken down (more or less completely) into amino acids. These smaller molecules (a little smaller than sugar molecules, they weigh roughly 100 times more than a hydrogen atom) are composed of carbon, hydrogen, oxygen, nitrogen, and sometimes sulfur. Along the "backbone" of a protein, the atoms nitrogen, carbon, and another carbon, from each amino acid, repeat regularly: NC-C, -N-C-C, -N-C-C, etc. The basic amine (ammonia-like) nitrogen at one end combines with the acidic carbon at the other end, and a variety of other atoms are attached to the middle carbon, as a "side-chain." The nature of the side chain is most important in determining the function of the protein. If the nitrogen is removed from the amino acid, what remains is a small acidic molecule, which in some cases is a common "fuel" molecule. Eight (roughly) of the 22 amino acids have a "carbon skeleton" which we can't synthesize, so they must be included in the diet — as protein, amino acid, or possibly as "skeleton."

Starch: a "macromolecule" consisting of strings of sugar molecules. They may be used for storage or for structural purposes, as in connective tissues. Glycogen is the storage starch of animals.

Sugar: a small carbohydrate, usually from 3 to 12 carbon atoms. An alcohol is intermediate between sugar and fat, usually with one or two oxygens per molecule.

Vitamins: any chemical which is necessary for life and has to be obtained in the diet, in small amounts — i.e., specific substances other than fuel molecules, protein (or amino acids) or minerals. The category includes, roughly, everything that's essential that doesn't fit another category. There is a popular tendency to give them the neat definition of "coenzymes," that is, a catalytic group other than a mineral which is associated with a protein to form a functional enzyme, and which can't be synthesized by the body — but unfortunately for that definition, some vitamins seem to have functions other than as co-enzymes. This mistaken definition often leads to the reasoning: "There are only so many molecules of each enzyme; therefore a similar number of vitamin molecules is the maximum that can be used." First, the number of enzyme molecules is variable; second, several factors can influence the association of co-enzyme with (apo)enzyme, so that there may be no effective "binding" until the protein is surrounded by a cloud of vitamin molecules; and third, the vitamin's function may not involve an enzyme at all. The "vitamin equals co-enzyme" concept seems to result from "quicky" biochemistry courses, combined with no study of nutrition.

UNITS OF MEASURE

The labels on vitamin bottles can be misleading to people who don't realize that a milligram (mg.) is 1000 times bigger than a microgram (mcg.). Usually the only vitamins that should be listed in microgram amounts are B12, biotin, and folic acid. For example, 50 mcg. of pantothenic acid is too small to do any good; it would be about the right dose for a big bug, but I have seen it on many vitamin labels. Apparently these are easy units to confuse — in one of my nutrition classes, a woman who had been a nurse for 30 years said she had always thought a microgram was bigger than a milligram.

The next larger common unit, the gram is easier to visualize: roughly a quarter of a teaspoonful, or about 1/28 of an ounce. One milligram is a thousandth of a gram. Sometimes the English unit, grain, is confused with the gram; a grain is abbreviated gr. (gram is g.) and is only about 65 milligrams.

Calories (or kilocalories) are the chemical energy of food expressed as heat, and for many foods the figures given in tables are misleading. For example, many vegetables contain carbohydrates with a variable digestibleness: storage or cooking can modify the amount that is available, and different people will absorb different proportions of them. The calorie values for fats (over 9 calories per gram) and carbohydrates (about 4 calories per gram) are more consistent. Chemically, protein has about 5 calories per gram, but this figure isn't very meaningful biologically. Taking "calories" out of context can give bad results — some people avoid carrots as being "high in calories," but carrots can be very effective for losing weight, partly because their high fiber content binds a large amount of fat and carries it out of the body. "International units" are used for vitamins A. D, and E. The minimum requirements for these vitamins are, in weight, close to those for vitamins B1, B12, and pantothenic acid, respectively. In international units, the figures are 5000 to 8000, about 400, and 25 to 30, but these requirements are known to vary with factors such as the amount of sunshine, the season, and other nutrients in the diet.

Vitamin A may also be expressed in the new unit, RE (retinol equivalent), which is 5 times as large as an IU.

NUTRIENTS: PLANT SOURCES; PLACES CONCENTRATED IN ANIMALS; FUNCTIONS

Vitamin A: leaves, carrots; eye, liver, skin; light sensitivity, protein synthesis, cell division regulation.

Vitamin K: leaves; liver; clotting, energy.

Vitamin D: milk products; teeth, bones, nerves, muscles; clotting — mineral metabolism.

Vitamin E: leaves, seeds; liver, fat, brain; energy, clot removal, cell integrity.

Vitamin B1: nuts, leaves, bran; liver, cornea; oxidative energy metabolism.

Niacin: nuts, seeds; liver; energy, synthesis.

Vitamin B6: leaves, fruit; meat in general; synthesis, especially proteins and nerve chemicals.

Biotin: seeds, leaves; liver, oviduct; synthesis of fats and oils, carbon dioxide metabolism.

Inositol: fruit, seeds, leaves; liver; mobilizing fats, stabilizing molecules and cells.

Vitamin B12: possibly in leaves, such as comfrey; pituitary gland, liver, other animal tissue; blood formation, nerve function, and it has been suggested for irregular menstruation and abnormal vaginal discharge.
Pantothenic acid: fruit, seeds; liver, glands; hormone production, energy, synthesis.
Folic acid: leaves, nuts; liver; synthesis, especially nerve, blood, immune system.
Vitamin C: fruits; glands; connective tissue, immunity, detoxification, anti-cholesterol.
Potassium: all solid parts; intracellular; lost in stress, deficiency mimics diabetes.
Sodium: saps especially; extracellular; well retained, except when adrenals are damaged or it is taken in excess.
Magnesium: leaves, molasses; intracellular; enzyme control, stabilizes nerves, muscles, etc. activates immune system, helps regulate sugar metabolism.
Calcium: milk, leaves; mainly extracellular; enzyme and permeability control, muscle contraction, clotting.
Phosphorous: seeds, yeast; meat, milk, intracellular; growth, energy, etc.
Iron: bran, molasses; blood, meat; respiration, enzymes.
Iodine: kelp. sea plants; all seafoods, thyroid gland; growth, fertility, nerve function, oxidation.
Copper: soy beans; liver; mitochondrial oxidation, elastin production in arteries, skin, etc., possible regulatory function in hormone cycles.
Zinc: sea plants; oysters, thymus gland; immunity, wound healing, fertility, nerves.
Ubiquinone: leaves; liver, all tissues; energy production, muscle action, acts with vitamin E.
Fiber: Carrot fibers are best for intestinal stimulation and binding of fats; leaves and bran contain fiber that is slightly less effective, though the other nutrients in them are very valuable.

Essential fatty acids: seeds, leaves; liver, pork, chicken; can prevent eczema; used in lecithin synthesis, and probably in prostaglandin hormones, kidney function.

HOLISTIC PHYSIOLOGY: A DIAGRAM

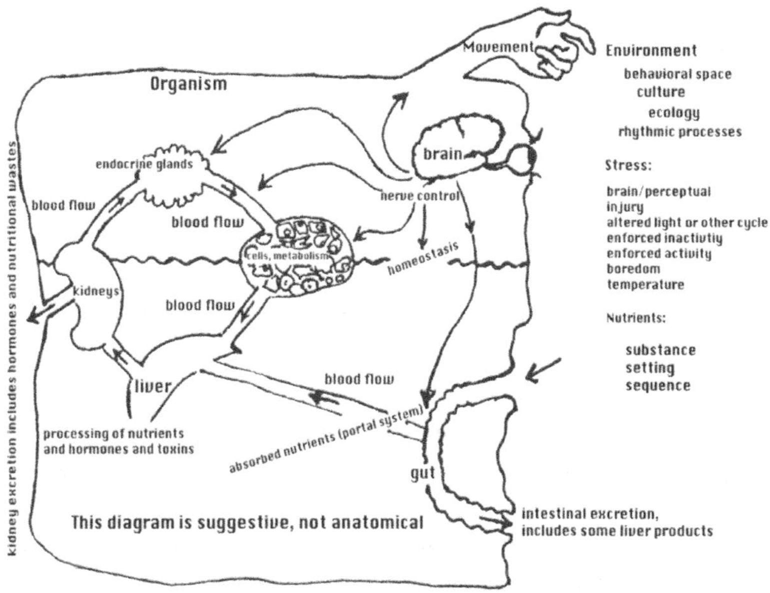

The wavy line across the middle of the picture represents the "internal environment," the fluid that bathes all our cells, which is kept as close as possible to an optimum composition. Water, salts, acid-alkali balance, hormones, sugars and other nutrients are all regulated as smoothly as possible. An abnormal environment can disturb the balance of one substance, and if the organism can't replace it from the environment or tissue stores, complex adjustment of many components can restore a reasonable balance. But the greater the demand, the smaller will be the reserve capacity for a future adaptation. Therefore, part of our "physiology" is the adjustment of our environment so that it more closely suits our needs. If our environment fails us a little today, our needs will be much greater tomorrow. For example, experiments show that if the cells of the cornea (eye surface) become deficient in vitamin B2, they can no longer pick up that vitamin from the body fluids when the animal is fed a normal amount of the vitamin. An extremely high dose must be given before the tissue can regain its normal amount of the vitamin. A similar effect has been observed with niacin, and it probably represents a general property of living material (physical systems show a similar effect. called hysteresis).

This kind of effect, this "residue" from past environments, has to be considered in deciding what a person's nutritional requirements are. Memory and intention must be considered as part of physiology: evaluating the quality of support from the environment requires a long time scale, even "transgenerational." Transgenerational effects are typically ignored or denied by establishment "science": A.E. Needham in *The Growth Process in Animals,* reviews some of the older studies of nutritional effects extending beyond a single lifetime. More recently, Zamenhof and others have shown transgenerational nutritional effects on the brain. Absolutist genetic theory — plus bad reasoning — serves to justify a given level of disease in the population. For example, nutritional standards are determined with reference to the present level of health in the nation, because this is seen as being determined by factors other than nutrition. The national health has deteriorated in many ways over the last 30 or 40 years, and the average diet has changed. Official national nutritional standards have been revised downward over this period.

Emphasizing the uniqueness of individual needs should be seen in the context of looking for the most general principles: this can help us to perceive meaningful configurations, making otherwise trivial things significant. I think a biophysical approach to the cytoplasm is one of the "principles" that will help in perceiving patterns. Other more specific and immediately useful ideas include stress, the use of sugar efficiently or wastefully. and the energy charge of cells. These are explained in other sections.

A NOTE ON REFERENCES

At present, Nutrition for Women contains more than 80 references to the scientific or medical literature. Since it is compactly written, almost every sentence is based on at least one publication. Complete citations would therefore require a bibliography at least as long as the present text, meaning that the book would cost more than twice as much. Often I have used older sources, when their results have stood up well, because I want to emphasize the cultural lag which exists between discovery and professional awareness and application. Unfortunately, some professional half-wits who have never read a scientific paper are able to point at the date of citation and say, "well, *now* we know better than this." This happens frequently in relation to the information on estrogen and iron, especially, even though many studies have appeared in recent months confirming the older data. The only real solution to this problem is to change our system of education and information distribution. However, if more detailed citations are needed for a particular problem I will be glad to provide them.

REFERENCES NOT GIVEN IN TEXT

Chatterjee, S. N., et al., **"Effect of intrauterine contraceptive suture on corpora lutes of guinea-pigs," Indian). Exp. Biol. 9: 105, 1971.**

Dove, G. E., et al., **"Oestrogenic function in postmenopausal women," I.** Reprod. Fert. 24: **18, 1971.**

Emerson, G. A. and H. M. Evans, "Restoration of fertility in successively older E-low female rats,"). Nutr. 18: **501, 1939.**

Frampton, J., "Increased oestrogen activity associated with postmenopausal bleeding," J. Obstet. Gyn. Br. Commonw. 73: **137, 1966.**

Gram, T. E. and I. R. Fouts, "Effect of alpha-tocopherol upon lipid peroxidation and drug metabolism in hepatic microsomes," Arch. Biochem. Biophys. 114: **331-335, 1966.**

Gyorgy, P., and C. S. Rose, "Tocopherol and hemolysis in vivo **and** in vitro," Ann. N. Y. Acad. Sci. 52: **231, 1949.**

Pous, D. L. and I. Comas, "La insuficiencia progestacional del endometrio," Proc. 3rd World Congr. Fert. Ster. **(Amsterdam): 593-595, 1959.**

Sanchez, A., et al., "Role of sugars in human neutrophilic phagocytosis," Am. J. Clin. Nutr. 26, **1180, 1973.**

J. S. Turner, The Chemical Feast, **Grossman, N. Y. 1970.**

Vitale, J.J., et al., **(mitochondria and magnesium), J. Biol.** Chem 228, **573, 1957.**

Schwarz, K., "Dietetic hepatic injuries and the mode of action of tocopherol," Ann. N. Y. Acad. Sci. 52: **225, 1949.**

Song, C. S. and A. Kappas, "The influence of estrogens, progestins, and pregnancy on the liver," Vitamins and Hormones 26: **147, 1968.**

Yokota, K. and Yamazaki, "Reaction of peroxidase with reduced nicotinamideadenine dinucleotide and reduced nicotinamide-adenine dinucleotide phosphate," Biochim. Biophys. Acta 105: 301-312, **1965.**

"Immune deficiency in malnutrition," Nutrition Reviews 33(11), **334, 1975.**

"New Evidence favors breast-feeding," Med. World News 16(13), 26, 1975.

"Thymic function in malnutrition," Nutrition Reviews 32(6), **100, 1974.**

"Ascorbic acid and the catabolism of cholesterol," Nutrition Reviews 31(5), **154, 1973.**

"The growth of children given stimulant drugs," Nutrition Reviews 31(3), **91, 1973.**

"Riboflavin and adrenal cortex," Nutrition Reviews 31(3), **95, 1973.**

"Maternal dietary supplementation and infant birth weight," Nutrition Reviews 31(2), **45, 1973.**

"Oral contraceptives and vitamin B6," Nutrition Reviews **31(2), 49, 1973. "Brain biochemistry and intrauterine growth,"** Nutrition Reviews 31(1), 16, 1973.

Other books, newsletters and articles by

Ray Peat available at:

www.raypeat.com

Made in the USA
Monee, IL
13 September 2026

62981016R00104